Angela Dowden BSc (
and Fellow of the Roya
writing and journalis
supplement industry,
She now writes on al
frequent contributor to the *Daily Mail and* ~~~~~~~~~~~~~~~~~~~~~~~~
and magazines.

Also available in Orion paperback

ARE YOU GETTING ENOUGH?

ANGELA DOWDEN

ORION

For my family and friends. Also for Smudge,
who nibbled the manuscript.

An Orion Paperback
First published in Great Britain in 1999 by
Orion Books Ltd, Orion House, 5 Upper St Martin's Lane,
London WC2H 9EA

A CIP catalogue record for this book
is available from the British Library.

ISBN: 0 75281 702 7

Printed and bound in Great Britain by
The Guernsey Press Co. Ltd, Guernsey, C.I.

CONTENTS

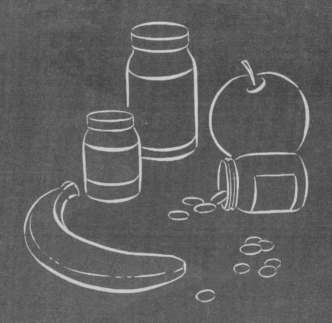

Are you getting enough vitamins and minerals? Fifty years ago a number of these nutrients had not even been discovered, much less become a part of every-day life. Now, one-third of us are popping vitamin pills or supplements in an attempt to counteract poor diet, make us healthier or ward off disease.

But should we really be so neurotic? Could worrying about what we eat actually do us more harm than anything else?

One thing that can't be disputed is that vitamins and minerals are essential to life. Our diet needs to provide us with a minimum amount of these nutrients, or even the most basic body processes like producing energy, using

> *vitamins and minerals are essential to life*

muscles and regulating our metabolic rate will suffer. And anything from missing out on vegetables to smoking can mean we become marginally deficient, with possible adverse effects on health.

Where the vitamin debate really starts is over the benefit – or otherwise – of doses above those officially recognised as preventing deficiency. An increasing amount of research shows that antioxidant vitamins, for example, may actually offer extra health benefits when taken at two, three or even ten times the normal recommended level.

Despite this, many orthodox health professionals insist that taking additional vitamins of any kind is a waste of money for healthy people. Meanwhile, the natural health experts claim that any self-help measure – including supplementation – with the potential to improve health and take the strain off the public purse should be strongly encouraged.

So what should we do? Popping a pill is not a panacea, but neither should *sensible* supplementation be ignored. In certain situations and for particular individuals, vitamins undoubtedly have a role in boosting vitamin and mineral intake and maintaining good health. In particular, groups like pregnant women, the elderly and children can benefit. But that said, the only *proven* message that scientists can give is that a healthy diet including five portions of fruits and vegetables a day – and not a handful of vitamins – is the key to optimum health.

The purpose of this book is not to say whether you should or should not take supplements. It provides you with the latest information on vitamins, minerals and a range of other factors so that you can make that decision for yourself. For each vitamin, mineral or supplement, information is given on functions, requirements and food sources, plus the benefits versus risks of higher dosages, and data on maximum safe intakes. Use the information as a way to increase your vitamin know-how, and to find out if you really are getting enough nutrients for your very best health.

> *Use the information as a way to increase your vitamin know-how*

CHAPTER 1

Introducing vitamins and minerals

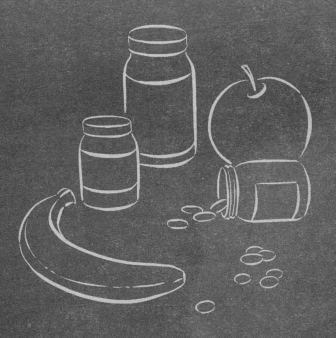

The food we eat is the key to life itself. Virtually every meal provides a combination of energy-giving carbohydrates, proteins for building and repairing body tissues, and fats for making vital cell membranes and helping to insulate the body. In addition to these 'macronutrients', nearly all foods provide much tinier quantities of 'micro-nutrients' – vitamins, minerals and trace elements. Despite their diminutive requirements, these nutri-ents are just as essential to our health as the macronutrients, and without them we can develop deficiency diseases and, in extreme cases, die.

The reason vitamins and minerals are so important is that they assist in the complex biochemical workings of the body. For example they help to regulate hormonal balance, lend strength to bones and assist in the function of nerves and muscles. Despite their popular 'pep-pill' image, vitamins and minerals do not in themselves supply any energy (calories), but they assist in many important energy-releasing reactions in the body. Without vitamins and minerals the efficient production of energy from macronutrients (carbohydrates, proteins and fats), would be impossible.

Vitamins and minerals can be distinguished from one another on the basis that vitamins are organic and minerals inorganic. Vitamins contain the vital elements carbon and hydrogen, and are largely manufactured by plants and bacteria. Minerals, on the other hand, originate in the earth's crust. They are taken up by plants, which are then eaten by animals – we can therefore obtain the minerals from either source. The similarity between

obtain a dietary supply to maintain health

vitamins and minerals is that humans must obtain a dietary supply of both to maintain health. We do not have the ability to make them ourselves.

VITAMINS

Thirteen substances have been classified as vitamins. These are vitamin A, vitamin D, vitamin E, vitamin K, vitamin C, thiamin (vitamin B1), riboflavin (vitamin B2), niacin (vitamin B3), pantothenic acid (vitamin B5), vitamin B6, folic acid, vitamin B12 and biotin. Beta carotene is a very important nutrient often referred to as a vitamin, but it does not officially have vitamin status.

The quantities of vitamins needed to prevent a deficiency are very small, varying from just one microgram to a few milligrams daily.

Vitamins can be subdivided into two groups: fat soluble and water soluble. Vitamins A, D, E and K are fat soluble which means that reserve supplies can be stored in the body. In theory, fat-soluble vitamins need not be consumed every day as the body can survive on its stores until a further top-up of the vitamin is supplied.

Vitamin C and the B complex are water soluble. Any excess of these vitamins is lost via the urine, and the body can only handle small intakes at one time. Water-soluble vitamins are ideally needed in regular daily amounts.

MINERALS

Around twenty to twenty-five minerals have so far been identified as essential for humans. These include calcium, phosphorus, iron, magnesium, zinc, iodine, copper, boron, chloride, chromium, manganese, molybdenum, nickel, potassium, selenium, silicon and sodium.

Sometimes the terms 'mineral' and trace element' are used interchangeably. However, 'mineral' or 'macromineral' is better used to describe the bulkier elements (calcium, phosphorus, magnesium, potassium, sodium and chloride) which are required in quantities greater than 100 milligrams per day, whereas 'trace element' or 'micromineral' more accurately describes those minerals which are needed in quantities less than 100 milligrams daily. A few, such as chromium, selenium and iodine, are needed in quantities less than one milligram daily and may occasionally be given the prefix 'ultra-trace'.

HOW VITAMINS AND MINERALS ARE MEASURED

The amounts of vitamins and minerals needed on a daily basis are tiny compared with the bulk of macronutrients we eat at each meal. On food labels and vitamin bottles you will see the quantities of vitamins or minerals given as weights, either milligrams (mg) or micrograms (μg or mcg). Comparison with the more familiar grams (g) will give some idea of their scale:

1 mg (one milligram)
   = 1/1000 g (one thousandth of a gram)
1 μg (one microgram)
   = 1/1000 mg (one thousandth of a milligram)
   or 1/1,000,000 g (one millionth of a gram)

To give an actual example, the daily requirement for calcium (a mineral needed in fairly 'large' amounts) is only equal to one-fifth the weight of a level teaspoon of sugar. The amount of vitamin B12 required on a daily basis is equivalent to less than a single grain of sand.

To confuse the matter of measurements further, vitamins A, D and E are also occasionally given in international units (IUs). International units express vitamins in terms of their biological activity rather than their weight. These older units were originally used before the vitamins could be purified and weighed. For comparison purposes, here are the conversions:

1 IU vitamin A = 0.3 μg
1 IU vitamin D = 0.025 μg
1 IU vitamin E = 0.67 mg

The amounts of vitamins and minerals needed on a daily basis are tiny

RECOMMENDED DAILY ALLOWANCES

Recommended Daily Allowances (RDAs) are often taken as literal requirements for vitamin and mineral intake. But if this were so then an American consuming 3 μg of vitamin B12 a day would be consuming an insufficient quantity of this nutrient, whereas a European taking the same amount would be obtaining triple the amount necessary for health! (B12: US RDA = 6μg, EU RDA = 1μg.)

In fact RDAs are scientific opinion (not fact), and at best can only be an estimate of the nutrient needs of a random population. They are pitched at the level sufficient to meet the basic vitamin and mineral needs of virtually all the population, and the same RDA can cover groups as diverse as sedentary office workers and heavy manual workers, who in reality may have very different individual vitamin requirements.

RDAs do not take into account the special nutritional needs that may occur through illness or genetic variation. More importantly, they do not reflect the level of a nutrient that may be needed for optimal health (see Optimum nutrition: a new concept, page 15).

sedentary office workers and heavy manual workers have different vitamin requirements

RDAS VS RNIS

Many variations of the RDA exist from country to country, with slightly different names and meanings. In 1991, the British Department of Health coined the phrase RNI (Reference Nutrient Intake) to replace the old Recommended Daily Amount and to remove the impression that RDAs are concrete 'recommendations' for individuals. To give a more accurate reflection of differing needs, RNIs were defined for both sexes and several age groups, as well as for pregnant and lactating mothers.

Some food labels and vitamin supplements give the percentage of the Recommended Daily Allowance provided by the product. In this case, the RDAs refer to a set of standardised EU RDAs used throughout the European Community for labelling purposes. There are twelve EU RDAs for vitamins and six for minerals. They are given in the following table, and are the RDAs routinely referred to throughout this book. A number of vitamins and minerals have not been given RDAs. This does not mean they are any less essential for the human body – it simply indicates there is less information on how much of these we need.

EU Recommended Daily Allowances

Vitamin	RDA	Mineral	RDA
Vitamin A (retinol)	800 µg	Calcium	800 mg
Vitamin B1 (thiamin)	1.4 mg	Iodine	150 µg
Vitamin B2 (riboflavin)	1.6 mg	Iron	14 mg
Vitamin B3 (niacin)	18 mg	Magnesium	300 mg
Vitamin B5 (pantothenic acid)	6 mg	Phosphorus	800 mg
Vitamin B6 (pyridoxine)	2 mg	Zinc	15 mg
Vitamin B12	1 µg		
Folic acid	200 µg		
Biotin	0.15 mg		
Vitamin C	60 mg		
Vitamin D	5 µg		
Vitamin E (tocopherol)	10 mg		

VITAMIN-RICH EATING

The most valuable way to obtain the vitamins and minerals your body needs is through eating a healthy, balanced diet. Food provides a large variety of nutritive and other components which promote health, and supplements can never replace this rich complexity.

Variety is the key to a vitamin-rich diet. Cereals, vegetables, fruit, bread, pasta, meat, fish and eggs all play an important part in meeting your nutrient needs, but they need to be eaten in the right proportions. Nutritionists split foods into five different groupings, and use the 'balance of good health' model to demonstrate the relative quantities of these that should be consumed.

> *Variety is the key to a vitamin-rich diet*

THE BALANCE OF GOOD HEALTH

Bread, other cereals and potatoes
Provide: B vitamins, various minerals.
Also: energy-giving starchy carbohydrates.
Aim for between five and eleven servings a day: one serving equates to a slice of bread, 3 tablespoons of breakfast cereal, 1 tablespoon of cooked rice or pasta or 2 smallish potatoes.

Fruit and vegetables
Provide: antioxidant vitamins (beta carotene, C and E).
Also: fibre and various phyto (plant) chemicals associated with reduced risk of disease.
Aim for at least five different servings of fruit and vegetables daily – fresh, frozen and canned count, including fruit juice and soup. A serving is approximately 75 g – that's around 3 table-spoons of peas, a standard sized serving of broccoli, a generous side salad or a small to medium apple.

Meat, fish and alternatives (beans, pulses, lentils, nuts)
Provide: iron, zinc, selenium, iodine, vitamin D, B vitamins.

Also: protein for the daily repair and renewal of tissues.

Eat two to three servings per day: one serving is around 75 g lean meat or skinless poultry, 140 g fish, 2 medium eggs (up to 6 a week) or 300 g cooked beans or lentils.

Milk and dairy foods

Provide: calcium, iodine, B vitamins, vitamins A and D.

Also: protein.

Eat two to three servings of dairy products daily: one serving equals 200 ml milk, a pot of yoghurt or a matchbox-size piece of cheese. Reduced-fat dairy products are higher in calcium but lower in fat-soluble vitamins (A and D) than full-fat ones.

Fatty and sugary foods

Provide: energy (calories), but few other nutrients.

In a balanced diet, chocolates and sweets, chips and crisps, biscuits, cakes, pastries, cream and ice cream should only feature occasionally, and should only be eaten in small amounts. Vegetable oils are important in the diet in small quantities. They provide vitamin E and essential fatty acids needed for healthy cell structure and hormone production.

CONSERVING VITAMINS AND MINERALS IN FOOD

Cooking and preparing food with proper care can significantly increase the amount of vitamins retained. Many vitamins are vulnerable to attack through heat, air, moisture and light. By contrast, minerals are quite stable, but can be leached away in cooking water. The following tips show how to preserve nutrients:

Buy fruit and vegetables as regularly as possible – they may already have been transported half way around the world and sat on the shop shelf for some time before being purchased. Store in a cool, dry place, or in the refrigerator, and eat within a few days. Frozen vegetables retain their vitamins well and are good choices, especially if you can only shop irregularly. Don't overlook canned fruits and vegetable either: these days, better

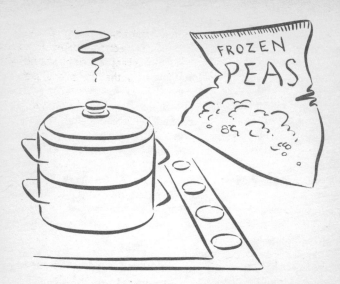

canning processes mean a higher percentage of nutrients is retained, and several varieties are now available without sugar and salt.

Think about how long you cook food

Cook vegetables for the minimum amount of time (so they are still crunchy). Steaming, quick stir-frying and microwaving are best at retaining vitamins. If you boil, use the minimum amount of water, introduce the vegetables straight to the hot water and use a tight-fitting lid. Pressure cooking is quicker but uses higher temperatures, so nutrient losses are about the same as boiling.

Think about how long you cook food. After twenty minutes of boiling, twenty per cent of the vitamin C in Brussels sprouts is lost. After thirty minutes, this figure rises to sixty-five per cent. Similarly, when rice is cooked in the minimum amount of water, thirty per cent of thiamin (vitamin B1) is lost, whereas when cooked in a large amount, fifty per cent is lost.

Frozen vegetables retain their vitamins well

> *Food standing for fifteen minutes may result in a twenty-five per cent loss of vitamin C*

Avoid leaving cut vegetables exposed to air, heat or light: cover them and chill. Don't soak prior to cooking, as the vitamins and minerals can dissolve away. Save cooking water and liquid from canned vegetables for making gravy, soup and sauces. And never use bicarbonate of soda to keep vegetables green – it completely destroys vitamin C.

When preparing fruit and vegetables it is best to cut or chop with a sharp knife rather than shred. Larger chunks rather than fine pieces will also lose less vitamins. Try to avoid peeling wherever possible as, in many cases, vitamins are most highly concentrated just under the skin.

Finally, once food is ready, try to eat it straight away because keeping it hot can destroy vitamins. Food standing for fifteen minutes may result in a twenty-five per cent loss of vitamin C, whilst food kept hot for ninety minutes, such as in a canteen, loses seventy-five per cent.

Storage/ handling/ cooking method	Vitamins likely to be destroyed
Exposure to bright light or sunlight	Riboflavin (e.g. in milk)
Cooking at high temperature e.g. canning	Vitamin A, beta carotene, folic acid, thiamin
Shelf storage	Vitamin C (diminishes with time), folic acid, vitamin E
Cooking in water	Vitamin C, riboflavin, niacin, thiamin, folic acid
Peeling vegetables	Vitamin C
Cooking with bicarbonate of soda	Vitamin C, thiamin
Shredding and slicing	Vitamin C, folic acid, vitamin E
Refining of grains (e.g. white flour)	Thiamin, niacin, vitamin E

HOW WELL DO WE REALLY EAT?

Although the theory is easy, it can be harder to eat a balanced diet in practice. With today's pace of life it is all too easy to skip meals, eat too much junk food, or miss out on nutrient-rich fruit and vegetables. Another problem is that, despite increasing rates of obesity, our calorie intakes have actually been falling. We are getting fatter, not through eating too much but by exercising too little.

The net result of eating fewer calories is that we may also achieve a poorer intake of vitamins and minerals. Of course, less active lifestyles also require less vitamins and minerals, but mental and emotional stresses can often replace the physical ones.

According to data on vitamin intake, women are at a higher risk of low intakes, perhaps because they eat less than men and are more likely to embark on restrictive slimming regimes. In the most recent major nutritional

> *women are at a greater risk of low intakes*

survey of vitamin and mineral intake in UK adults, the risk of deficiency in the population as a whole was very small. But for women of child-bearing age, there were some notable exceptions (see following table).

Although, these days, people don't keel over and die of vitamin deficiencies like scurvy or beri-beri, they may suffer sub-clinical deficiencies which can undermine health in the long term. As well as menstruating women, groups most at risk include the elderly, slimmers, children and teenagers (especially faddy eaters), people on restricted diets (e.g. coeliacs or people with a dairy intolerance), strict vegetarians and hard-training athletes. These are the people most liable to benefit from supplementing their diet with a daily multivitamin or choosing fortified foods, such as breakfast cereals.

Some examples of low vitamin and mineral intakes in females aged 16–54*

Nutrient	Recommended Daily Allowance/ Reference Nutrient Intake	Actual Average Intake From Food (per day)
Magnesium	300 mg/270 mg	237 mg

Comments The average intake of this mineral is lower than recommended. Magnesium is important in energy release and for the nervous system.

Vitamin E	10 mg/none exists	7.2 mg

Comments On average, intake of this important antioxidant falls below the RDA. 2.5 per cent of women are estimated to achieve an intake of less than 3 mg a day – regarded as the absolute minimum to be safe.

Iron	14 mg/14.8 mg	12.3 mg

Comments Iron is needed to prevent anaemia, but the the average intake (including from supplements) is just 12.3 mg a day. From food alone, the average intake is only 10.5 mg. The worst dietary intakes of all are in the 16–24 age group.

Vitamin B6	2 mg/1.2 mg	1.57 mg

Comments Average vitamin B6 intake is borderline. Low intakes may be compounded by the contraceptive pill which can deplete B6 from the body.

Calcium	800 mg/700 mg	726 mg

Comments Again intakes are borderline. Fifty per cent of women consume less than 716 mg calcium daily, while 2.5 per cent have less than 268 mg daily.

*The Dietary and Nutritional Survey of British Adults (HMSO, 1990)

OPTIMUM NUTRITION: A NEW CONCEPT

Could it be that vitamins consumed in *excess* of the RDA hold the key to even better health? Years ago such an idea would have been preposterous to nutritional scientists, but increasingly it seems likely to be true. For example the *American Journal of Clinical Nutrition* recently suggested that 200 mg vitamin C daily would be a more desirable figure for maintaining consistently high tissue levels of this nutrient than the traditional RDA of 60 mg. In this case, the higher level can easily be obtained through dietary means – 200 mg is the amount in just two large glasses of orange juice.

In other cases – for example folic acid – the higher levels now known to promote optimum reproductive health are rarely achievable through normal diet alone. Without supplementation, women of child-bearing age cannot easily achieve the amount of folic acid they need to give maximum protection against birth defects, so individuals planning a child or in the early stages of pregnancy must take a 400 μg tablet of folic acid in addition to what they obtain through food.

Similarly, with vitamin E, 10 mg (the RDA) is enough for vital functions such as normal growth and development, but around seven to ten times this may be needed to protect against heart disease, especially in vulnerable groups.

PLAYING SAFE

With more and more studies hinting that vitamins might stave off disease, it's tempting to shove a handful down your gullet double quick. But optimising nutrition doesn't mean willy-nilly self-supplementation with megadose

too many vitamins in the wrong combination can be as harmful as too few

vitamin cocktails – too many vitamins in the wrong combination can be as harmful as too few.

In the now famous Finnish study, published in 1994, high doses of beta carotene given to lifelong heavy smokers had the

> *know your safe limits and stick to them*

effect of marginally *increasing*, not decreasing, lung cancer risk. It is now realised that a high dose of beta carotene may change from being antioxidant (protective) to pro-oxidant (damaging) in the presence of low levels of vitamin C – which are very common in heavy smokers. In fact, in several cases, high doses of individual nutrients can unbalance others with negative effects. For example excessive zinc can reduce the level of copper in the body, and large amounts of calcium can inhibit the absorption of iron.

KNOW YOUR LIMITS

So vitamins should be treated with respect. In the past, attempts to avoid overdosing with vitamin and mineral supplements meant tying the maximum recommended intake to a multiple of the RDA. But latest evidence shows this approach is arbitrary and unscientific. That's because each vitamin and mineral has its own margin of safety. For example, vitamin E at daily intakes up to eighty times higher than the RDA are quite safe; whereas in the case of zinc, long-term supplemental intakes may be undesirable at only a little over the RDA.

The really smart way to take supplements is to know your safe limits and stick to them. In recent years, the vitamin industry has invested heavily in independent research to establish maximum safe levels for self-supplementation. The conclusions of this research – published by the European Federation of Health Product Manufacturers – are given in the table below, and now form the basis of a voluntary self-policing policy for the vitamin industry. The Upper Safe Levels indicate amounts that have never been reported to harm a healthy person. If you are concerned you may be overdoing your vitamins, you should check the labels and make sure your total intake does not exceed the figures given.

Daily Upper Safe Levels of supplement intake

Nutrient	Upper Safe Level* (long term)	Upper Safe Level (short term)
Vitamin A	2300 µg (maximum 800 µg during pregnancy)	7500 µg
Vitamin D	10 µg	50 µg
Vitamin E	800 mg	>800 mg
Vitamin C	2000 mg	3000 mg
Thiamin	100 mg	100 mg
Riboflavin	200 mg	200 mg
Nicotinic acid**	150 mg	500 mg
Niacinamide	450 mg	1500 mg
Vitamin B6	100 mg	200 mg
Folic acid	400 µg	700 µg
Vitamin B12	3000 µg	3000 µg
Biotin	2.3 mg	2.5 mg
Pantothenic acid	1000 mg	1000 mg
Beta carotene	20 mg	>20 mg
Calcium	1500 mg	1900 mg
Phosphorus	1500 mg	1500 mg
Iron	15 mg	80 mg
Magnesium	300 mg	400 mg
Zinc	15 mg	50 mg
Iodine	500 µg	700 µg
Manganese	15 mg	20 mg
Molybdenum	200 µg	10,000 µg
Selenium	200 µg	700 µg
Copper	5 mg	8 mg
Chromium	200 µg	300 µg

*The Upper Safe Levels are designed for self-supplementation. They may be exceeded on the advice of a health professional.
**Niacinamide (nicotinamide) and nicotinic acid are two versions of niacin (vitamin B3). Nicotinic acid is not as safe in large quantities as niacinamide. This table assumes that one or the other form is taken, not both (check ingredients list on label).

CHAPTER 2

Choosing and using supplements

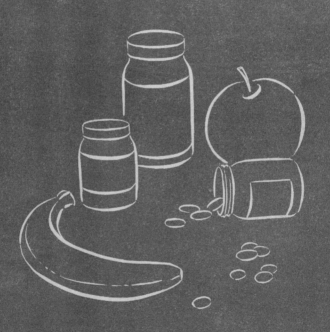

*S*uppose you decide to start taking a vitamin supplement. It sounds simple in theory, but in practice there's a baffling choice. Just walk into any pharmacy or health food store and you'll be faced with a sea of supplements from A to zinc and everything in between.

WHICH SUPPLEMENT/ WHAT DOSAGE?

First, check if you have an obvious vitamin or mineral requirement with our quick 'Are you getting enough?' quiz in chapter eight. Chapter six, on special vitamin needs, also gives an indication of what your supplement needs might be.

Baffled by the range of dosages available?

Baffled by the range of dosages available? For preventing deficiencies, every-day nutritional insurance and maintenance of health, a basic, lower potency product is perfectly suitable. To help *treat* a deficiency, improve certain aspects of your health or relieve an ailment, you may need a top-end supplement with a higher potency. Bear in mind that you should always keep within the Upper Safe Levels given in chapter one, unless specifically advised by a health professional.

UNDERSTANDING THE LABEL

Most vitamin and mineral products are legally classified and labelled as foods. The packaging must carry various key pieces of information, including an ingredients box, a lot number and a best-before date. Although labels can vary in their precise layout, the following is a typical example:

MR STRONGBONE'S CALCIUM COMPLEX – 90 TABLETS

Ingredients: [1] Calcium carbonate, Magnesium oxide, Zinc gluconate, Manganese gluconate, vitamin D compound…etc.
Directions: Swallow two tablets twice daily. [2]
Nutrition information – typical values:

	Per two tablets [3]	%RDA [4]
Vitamin D	2.5µg	50
Calcium	400 mg	50
Magnesium	150 mg	50
Zinc	5 mg	33
Manganese	2 mg	– [5]

Keep out of the reach of children. [6]
Store tightly closed in a cool, dry place. [7]
LOT: [8]   Best before end:[9]
Mr Strongbone's Vitamin Company, Any Street, Any Town, UK.[10]

---

(1) All ingredients are listed in descending weight order. This includes nutrients and non-active ingredients (excipients) used to formulate the supplement.

(2) These are the manufacturer's recommended usage instructions.

(3) Nutritional information is given per quantified amount of the supplement to be taken at any one time – in this case per two tablets.

(4) This indicates the percentage of the EU Recommended Daily Allowance provided by the nutrient (on supplements for adults and children over four years).

(5) Some nutrients have not been designated an RDA.

(6) All supplements, particularly iron, should be kept out of the reach of children.

(7) Follow the storage instructions carefully. Supplements should generally be kept in a cool, dry place in the original container.

(8) All products must bear a lot or batch number for full traceability.

(9) The product should be used before the 'best before' date to assure full potency.

(10) The manufacturer's, or distributor's, name and address are required to appear on the label.

CHOOSING A MULTIVITAMIN

In fact, for the majority of people who take supplements, a multivitamin is most appropriate to their needs. A good multivitamin can make up for any minor nutrient shortfalls in your diet, and may also help boost your body's defences against infections and minor illnesses. A study published in the *Lancet* in 1992 found that a regular multivitamin and mineral supplement improved the functioning of the immune system and reduced the risk of infection in older people.

A multivitamin will contain a range of vitamins, and often, though not always, some minerals. The most basic products only include small amounts of a narrow selection of nutrients (e.g. vitamins A, C, D, E and calcium). For a less hit-and-miss approach, plump for a multivitamin containing at least the Recommended Daily Allowance of a wider selection of nutrients. A number of these more comprehensive one-a-day formulations are now on the market, retailing at less than the price of a daily newspaper.

Don't be taken in by fancy packaging or an ingredients list as long as your arm. There are only so many 'extras' you can pack into a supplement before you start diluting the amounts of valuable nutrients that really *are* needed by the body. Many ingredients are not vital nutrients, but are added (usually in insignificant amounts) purely for marketing purposes, and to make the product seem 'healthier' than it really is.

> *A good multivitamin can make up for any minor nutrient shortfalls in your diet*

A MINERAL MINEFIELD

Most minerals exist naturally as mineral salts, e.g. iron oxide – the major constituent of iron ore. Arguments rage over the best forms of mineral salts for supplements, but on the whole, organic salts – which contain a chain of carbon atoms – are thought to be better absorbed than inorganic salts, although there may be individual exceptions. Organic salts include lactates, fumerates, malates, citrates and gluconates; inorganic salts include chlorides, sulphates, oxides and carbonates.

Amino acid chelated minerals have been hailed as the gold standard for supplements. These are minerals which have been bound with the building blocks of proteins: specific examples include zinc picolinate and selenomethionine (selenium bound with the amino acid methionine). Amino acid chelates have definitely proved to be more effectively absorbed in animals, but little testing has been done on humans.

Providing you have a good digestion and you take your supplement with a meal, the form of the minerals shouldn't matter. But for older people, or people with poor digestion or low stomach acid, one of the more sophisticated mineral forms could be better.

TIMED-RELEASE PREPARATIONS

Because water-soluble B and C vitamins cannot be stored in the body, a sudden high influx can super-saturate the system leading to the loss of these nutrients via the urine.

Higher-dose supplements may therefore be presented in a slow-release form (also known as sustained release, timed release or prolonged release). Slow-release tablets are formulated to gradually release their nutrients for absorption over a period of around six to eight hours. They need to be taken with food to work properly.

The alternative to timed-release vitamins is taking smaller doses more frequently.

TABLET, CAPSULE OR LIQUID?

Supplements are available in all sorts of different guises. What you choose is down to personal preference, but here's a rundown which might help you decide:

Capsules are generally made with gelatin and can be hard (made of two pieces and usually containing powders) or pliable (filled with liquid or paste). Two-piece capsules may also be pulled apart and the powder taken separately.
Pros: Capsules usually contain fewer excipients (non-active ingredients) than tablets. They are generally easier to swallow than equivalent tablet formulations and are easily digested.
Cons: Gelatin is made from animal bones and therefore not suitable for vegetarians or vegans. However some starch or seaweed-based alternatives are becoming available and are worth looking out for if you prefer to avoid gelatin.

Tablets are made by mixing together all the relevant powder ingredients and compressing these into a tablet using very high pressures.
Pros: Many tablet formulations are suitable for vegetarians and vegans. Tablets are also relatively less expensive than comparable hard and soft gelatin capsules.
Cons: Some people don't find tablets as easy to swallow as capsules.

Chewable tablets are commonly used for children's formulations, and are also often used for calcium, multivitamin and vitamin C products.
Pros: Pleasant to take, and you can take them without water. Good if you can't swallow tablets or capsules.
Cons: Can contain high levels of sugar or sweetener which some users might find unacceptable.

Liquids are a more traditional supplement form, used for iron preparations, cod liver oil, vitamin tonics, etc.
Pros: Easily assimilated, and suitable for people who cannot

swallow tablets or capsules.
Cons: It may be difficult to control dosage unless a proper measuring spoon is used. Liquids in bottles are not very portable.

Effervescent tablets are a common way of providing vitamin C and other nutrients.
Pros: Pleasant way of taking the nutrient.
Cons: Expensive; the tablets may also contain sweeteners, flavourings and other unnecessary additives.

DOES TIMING MATTER?

What time of day should you take vitamins? Many people think it should be in the morning, but exactly when is on the whole unimportant. What matters more is establishing a daily routine so that you don't forget your vitamins one day and then take too many the next.

Unless the label specifically states otherwise, it is best to take supplements with a meal as they function in combination with the vitamins and minerals in food. Tablets and capsules should also be swallowed with plenty of water to ensure the best absorption.

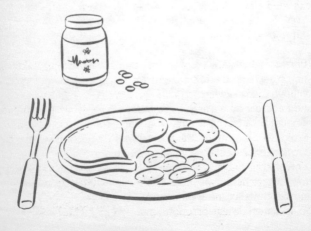

ARE NATURAL VITAMINS BETTER?

Despite the marketing hype surrounding 'natural' supplements, most vitamins are absorbed and utilised by the body in exactly the same way regardless of their source. For example, ascorbic acid (vitamin C) is the same whether it is synthesised in a manufacturing plant or comes from an orange.

Vitamin E is the only vitamin that is less active, weight for weight, when it is synthetically made. Manufactured vitamin E is known as dl-tocopherol and is a mixture of eight compounds; vitamin E derived from a natural source (normally soya oil) is a single entity called d-alpha tocopherol, and possesses a higher biological activity.

most vitamins are absorbed and utilised by the body in exactly the same way regardless of their source

To ensure consistency between products, the labelling regulations require that the potency of vitamin E stated on the label always refers to the d-alpha tocopherol equivalent. However, current labelling rules only account for a 36 pc potency difference between d- and dl-alpha tocopherol and recent studies indicate natural vitamin E may actually be twice as effective.

SUPPLEMENT QUALITY

There is much debate over the status of vitamins sold as supplements. In the UK, as long as these supplements do not break food law – which requires that they be safe, wholesome and free from false claims – they can be freely sold. But should they continue to be so freely available, or be reclassified as medicines and more tightly regulated? According to the Consumers' Association, forty per cent of consumers already believe that supplements are medicines, and yet there are no legal controls on maximum dosage or reporting of

buy from a reputable source

adverse effects. The association wants all supplements to be subject to independent scrutiny before being marketed, with only approved claims being made for products.

In the future, it is likely that supplements will be given their own regulatory category, and the European Union has been drawing up proposals to this end. This could have certain advantages and help ensure quality, but manufacturers and some consumers are worried that it might restrict the availability of higher dosages. In many other European countries it is illegal to sell vitamins at doses much above the RDA unless the product is prescribed by a doctor or sold by a pharmacist.

Whatever the future for supplements, unfortunately there will probably always be a small minority of fly-by-night companies willing to dupe or offer false hope to consumers through offering poorly labelled products or making false claims (e.g. 'cures cancer', 'helps weight loss', etc.).

The best advice is always to buy from a reputable source, and avoid 'too good to be true' offers: they usually are!

CHAPTER 3
Vitamins

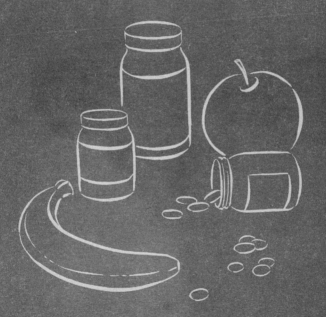

VITAMIN A

Vitamin A (retinol) is a fat-soluble vitamin which only occurs naturally in animal foods. It accumulates in the liver, so high doses can be toxic.

> *Vitamin A really can help us see in the dark!*

The RDA is 800 µg, but because it can be stored, larger amounts of the vitamin can be consumed less frequently.

WHAT DOES IT DO?
Vitamin A really can help us see in the dark! It is an important component of visual purple, which is essential for night-time vision. The vitamin also bolsters our immune defences, and is vital for the health of protective mucous surfaces found in the respiratory tract, vagina and gut. Vitamin A helps the skin maintain its natural oil layer and can also help prevent spots and infection.

WHERE IS IT FOUND?
The very best sources of vitamin A are cod liver oil, liver and kidney. Lesser amounts are found in butter, full-fat dairy products and margarine, oily fish and eggs. The vitamin may also be obtained from the conversion of carotenoids in richly coloured fruits and vegetables such as carrots, spinach and cantaloupe melons. This conversion is inefficient (6 µg beta carotene are converted to 1 µg vitamin A) but represents a very valuable supply of the vitamin for vegetarians.

ARE YOU GETTING ENOUGH?
To supply the RDA of vitamin A you would need to eat just 4 g lamb's or pig's liver, OR 100 g butter, OR 1.5 l whole-fat milk, OR 67 g carrots. Requirements are increased further during breast-feeding. True deficiency of vitamin A is rare, but signs and symptoms include rough, hardened skin, night blindness and increased susceptibility

> *Slimmers or people following very low-fat diets are most likely to lack the vitamin*

to infections. Slimmers or people following very low-fat diets are most likely to lack the vitamin, and multivitamins or cod liver oil are the most convenient way of taking it in supplement form.

PLAYING SAFE
Chronic intakes in excess of around 7500 μg vitamin A daily can cause headaches, fatigue, painful bones, loss of appetite and dry and scaly skin conditions. High doses may also cause birth defects, so eating liver, or taking supplements containing more than the RDA (800 μg) during pregnancy is not recommended. For everyone else, the maximum safe supplement intake is 2300 μg per day, or 7500 μg in the short term.

BETA CAROTENE

Beta carotene is the primary member of a family of plant pigments called carotenoids. Because there is not a specific deficiency disease associated with a low intake of beta carotene it is technically not a vitamin, and consequently there is no RDA. Nevertheless there is an increasing amount of evidence to support the role of beta carotene and other carotenoids in promoting health.

WHAT DOES IT DO?
One of beta carotene's roles is as a backup vitamin A supply. If the body falls short of this vitamin, beta carotene can be diverted into its manufacture, but the conversion is inefficient (see under Vitamin A section).

More importantly, beta carotene and other carotenoids act in their own right as antioxidants – factors that mop up highly reactive free radicals which, in excess, can damage body cells and tissues. Many studies have shown that a low blood level of beta carotene predicts a higher future risk of cancer, so a good dietary intake of beta carotene over the long term may be important in preventing this disease. However 'magic bullet' beta carotene supplements cannot undo the damage of a life-time's exposure to free radicals, and may even be counterpro-ductive. In a Finnish study published in 1994, the incidence of lung cancer was slightly increased in lifelong heavy smokers who took high-dose beta carotene supplements.

Research also shows an association between beta carotene and cardiovascular disease. In one study involving 1500 men under the age of seventy, there was a strong link between high consumption of dietary beta carotene and reduced risk of heart attack. And in a subgroup of heart patients from the famous US Physicians health study, beta carotene supplements reduced the risk of subsequent coronary events by fifty per cent.

In addition, there is some evidence that supplements of beta carotene nutrient may help improve the effectiveness of sunscreens; for many years high intakes of beta carotene have been used as a medication to treat severe sun sensitivity.

WHERE IS IT FOUND?

One of the richest sources of beta carotene is carrots. Good supplies of carotenoids in general can be found in all richly coloured fruits and vegetables, especially spinach, broccoli, cantaloupe melons, tomatoes, red peppers, mangoes and sweet peppers.

ARE YOU GETTING ENOUGH?

Although there is no EU RDA for beta carotene intake, antioxidant experts estimate that a figure of around 6 mg is probably a desirable daily intake. This is the amount in 75 g of carrots, OR 200 g cantaloupe melon, OR 460 g Brussels sprouts. Unfortunately, the average amount most of us achieve in our diets is only around 2–2.5 mg per day, with lowest levels usually in smokers. To achieve a more adequate intake we should all aim to eat at least least five varied portions of fruits and vegetables each day.

PLAYING SAFE

There are no direct toxic effects from overdosing on beta carotene, but more than about 20–30 mg daily can cause a reversible yellowing of the skin. There is also concern that high-dose beta carotene supplements (20 mg or more) can have an adverse effect in heavy smokers, perhaps through unbalancing other antioxidants in the body. Scientists now believe that beta carotene interacts in a positive way with other antioxidants, so if you want to take a supplement, keep safe by choosing one that provides beta carotene in conjunction with other nutrients in a low to moderate dose. Supplements derived from Dunaliella salina may be a particularly good choice as they contain natural beta carotene in combination with a small amount of other carotenoids.

VITAMIN B1 (THIAMIN)

Thiamin is a water-soluble nutrient and the first member of the B complex. The RDA for the vitamin is 1.4 mg.

WHAT DOES IT DO?
Thiamin is vitally important for the release of energy from carbohydrates, fat and alcohol. It also aids in the functioning of the nervous system and in nerve transmission.

Some people take high doses of thiamin to deter biting insects. It is believed that the 'smell' of the vitamin through the skin can help keep bugs at bay, although this hasn't been proven and certainly doesn't work for everybody.

WHERE IS IT FOUND?
Thiamin is found in foods such as whole grains, meat and fish (especially pork), milk, nuts, pulses and fortified breakfast cereals.

ARE YOU GETTING ENOUGH?
The RDA of thiamin is supplied by 140 g cornflakes, OR 160 g lean roast pork, OR approximately 11 slices wholemeal bread. People who have high-sugar diets or who drink a lot of alcohol have higher needs for the vitamin. Stress also uses it up at a faster rate. Beri-beri is the classical thiamin deficiency disease (symptoms include confusion, muscle weakness, enlarged

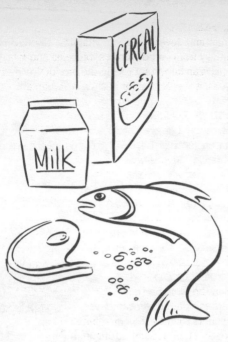

heart), but it is rare in the UK except amongst alcoholics. However, minor deficiencies, causing symptoms such as irritability, minor depression and weight loss are possible in people with a generally poor diet. They may benefit from a multivitamin or B-complex supplement in conjunction with dietary changes.

PLAYING SAFE

Thiamin is one of the safest known vitamins. There are no known side effects from taking high amounts, but the maximum level in supplements is voluntarily limited to 100 mg.

VITAMIN B2 (RIBOFLAVIN)

Riboflavin is a yellow-coloured, water-soluble nutrient and the second member of the B complex. The RDA for the vitamin is 1.6 mg.

WHAT DOES IT DO?
Like thiamin and several other B vitamins, riboflavin helps to release energy from carbohydrates, proteins and fats. The vitamin also plays an important role in the production and repair of body tissues: it is essential for healthy hair, skin and nails.

WHERE IS IT FOUND?
Riboflavin is found in good supply in liver and kidney. It is also present in other meats, full-fat and skimmed dairy products, fortified cereals and yeast extract.

ARE YOU GETTING ENOUGH?
Eating 90 g lamb's kidney, OR 70 g Shreddies, OR 900 ml milk, OR 15 g Marmite (enough for a thick scraping on four pieces of bread), will provide the RDA of riboflavin. The vitamin is destroyed by the action of light, so don't leave bottles of milk standing on the doorstep.

riboflavin is essential for healthy hair, skin and nails

Deficiencies of riboflavin can cause oral complaints such as sore, burning lips, mouth ulcers and tongue ailments. The eyes can also be affected, with burning and itchiness. Severe deficiency is very rare but minor shortfalls can occur in the diets of vegans who avoid all animal products, including dairy produce. Smoking, heavy drinking and the contraceptive pill may also increase the chance of deficiency.

PLAYING SAFE
Like thiamin, riboflavin is also a safe vitamin. In studies, high levels have not been associated with any side effects, probably because excesses are lost in the urine. If you take very high doses of riboflavin, you may notice that your urine becomes a bright yellow or green colour. This is actually harmless, but you will probably want to lower the amount you take. Most supplement companies stick to a voluntary maximum of 100 mg in supplements.

VITAMIN B3 (NIACIN)

Niacin is an unusual member of the B complex in that it can withstand heating and storage with minimal loss. Two slightly different forms of the vitamin exist – niacinamide and nicotinic acid – but niacin is the blanket term for both. Niacin can also be made in the body from an amino acid (protein building block) called tryptophan. Sixty molecules of niacin are needed to make just one molecule of niacin: the exception is during pregnancy when this conversion becomes a lot more efficient. The RDA for niacin is 18 mg.

WHAT DOES IT DO?

Like its partners, thiamin and riboflavin, niacin works to help release energy from food. It is one of the essential 'cogs' in the energy-releasing cycle that is at work in our cells every minute of the day and night. It also helps maintain healthy nerves. In very high doses the nicotinic acid form of niacin acts as a cholesterol-lowering drug, but there can be side effects, such as flushing and liver enlargement. Supplements of niacinamide have been claimed to help osteoarthritis, but there is little evidence to confirm this.

WHERE IS IT FOUND?

The best sources of niacin are fortified breakfast cereals and all types of meat and fish. Whole grains, pulses, nuts and, to a lesser extent dairy products, also supply reasonable amounts.

niacin helps maintain healthy nerves

ARE YOU GETTING ENOUGH?

The RDA for niacin can be supplied by a medium boneless chicken breast, OR 100 g peanuts, OR 780 g boiled spaghetti, OR 2 l milk. Most people get more than enough niacin in their diets, although alcoholics may become deficient and breastfeeding women need to increase their intakes to meet higher needs. Signs of a minor shortfall include tiredness and depression. The more severe deficiency disease, pellagra, (characterised by dermatitis, diarrhoea and dementia) is very rare in the UK.

PLAYING SAFE

Because of concerns over liver damage, timed-release nicotinic acid supplements have been withdrawn from sale in the UK. The European Federation of Health Product Manufacturers says that for long-term use supplements of non-timed-release nicotinic acid are safe up to 150 mg daily, and that niacinamide is safe up to 450 mg daily. In practice no more than 50–100 mg niacin is normally present in supplements, and nutritionally there can be no reason for wanting to exceed this level of intake. Large doses of niacin are unsuitable for people with diabetes, gout, stomach ulcers or liver disease.

VITAMIN B5 (PANTOTHENIC ACID)

Pantothenic acid is a water-soluble B-complex vitamin. It is widely available in the diet (*panthos* means 'everywhere' in Greek), and is sometimes known as the 'anti-stress' vitamin. The RDA for pantothenic acid is 6 mg.

WHAT DOES IT DO?

Pantothenic acid works with other B vitamins in metabolising carbohydrates, proteins and fats. It is a constituent of coenzyme A, an important part of the energy-releasing cycle in all body cells. The vitamin also helps in the manufacture of antibodies, which are needed to fight invading bacteria in our bodies.

In addition, pantothenic acid is required for the formation of cortisone – the hormone that enables the body to handle stress. Cortisone has a mild anti-inflammatory effect, and some rheumatoid arthritis sufferers therefore take extra pantothenic acid to help cope with the disease. One study using very

> *Pantothenic acid is sometimes known as the 'anti-stress' vitamin*

large doses (500 mg pantothenic a day for eight weeks) didn't alter the course of the disease, but did help pain and stiffness.

Sometimes pantothenic acid is also advocated for relieving stress or helping with allergies, but there is no strong evidence to support these uses.

WHERE IS IT FOUND?
Pantothenic acid is found in a wide variety of foods, but especially in liver, kidney, other meats, eggs, peanuts, oranges and potatoes.

ARE YOU GETTING ENOUGH?
You can obtain the RDA of pantothenic acid from 75 g lamb's liver, OR 350 g peanuts, OR 9 boiled eggs, OR 7 baked potatoes, OR 15 oranges. Because all foods contain a small amount, it is not normally lacking in our diets, but alcoholics and those using long-term antibiotics may need extra. Stress may also create an increased need for the vitamin. There are no clear deficiency symptoms.

PLAYING SAFE
Pantothenic acid is a very safe vitamin with no known toxic effects. In supplements it may be present at levels up to 500 mg, but lower levels (as part of a B-complex or multivitamin formulation) are much more common.

VITAMIN B6 (PYRIDOXINE)

Vitamin B6 is another important member of the water-soluble B complex. It is sometimes called the 'anti-depression' vitamin. The RDA for vitamin B6 is 2 mg.

WHAT DOES IT DO?
The vitamin is needed for the metabolism of proteins in the body, and also helps the nervous system in a number of ways. It is required for the production of serotonin, a brain chemical affecting mood, behaviour and sleep patterns.

High levels of vitamin B6 are sometimes used as a treatment

for premenstrual syndrome (PMS). Evidence for a beneficial effect is inconclusive, but one study involving 630 women at St Thomas's hospital, London, showed good results for many women after supplementing with 40–200 mg vitamin B6 on a regular basis.

the 'anti-depression' vitamin

In some sufferers with low vitamin B6 levels 100–200 mg vitamin B6 taken daily for at least three months has also been effective in preventing the progression of 'carpal tunnel syndrome' – inflammation of the nerve as it passes through the wrist. There are also reports that vitamin B6 can help reduce asthma symptoms and may help treat pregnancy nausea.

WHERE IS IT FOUND?
The best sources of vitamin B6 include fortified breakfast cereals, fish, liver, bananas, avocados and potatoes.

ARE YOU GETTING ENOUGH?
The RDA of vitamin B6 is provided by 100 g Special K, OR 4 avocados, OR 540 g poached cod, OR 7 bananas. Alcohol can deplete levels of vitamin B6 as can the asthma drug, theophylline, and oestrogen therapy (HRT or the contraceptive pill).

PLAYING SAFE
All experts agree that high levels of Vitamin B6 can cause nerve damage (with symptoms such as pins and needles, tingling and numbness), but the safe limit is strongly disputed. In 1997 the government put forward plans to restrict the maximum level allowable in a supplement (apart from those sold by a pharmacist or prescribed by a GP) to 10 mg. However, the public outcry, together with new evidence from scientists, forced them to back down. The current consensus among experts seems to be that up to 200 mg daily is in fact safe.

People taking the Parkinson's disease medication, levadopa, should avoid vitamin B6 supplements as the vitamin can reverse the effects of the drug.

VITAMIN B12

Vitamin B12 is another member of the B complex, and is some-times called 'anti-pernicious factor' because of its ability to prevent the condition pernicious anaemia. The absorption of vitamin B12 is helped by a substance called intrinsic factor which is secreted in gastric juices. The EU RDA for vitamin B12 is just 1 μg, but in other countries, recommended intakes are higher than this.

WHAT DOES IT DO?

The functions of vitamin B12 and another B vitamin – folic acid – are closely linked. The vitamins are involved together in the production of new cells, in particular red blood cells. Vitamin B12 also helps in nervous function and is required for the health of the myelin sheath – a protective casing around nerve fibres which speeds up the passage of nerve transmissions. For this reason, the vitamin is sometimes taken in high doses by people with multiple sclerosis, although there is no strong evidence that it helps.

According to research carried out at Trinity College in Ireland, vitamin B12 may help reduce the risk of birth defects. Folic acid is better known for this function, but researchers at the Dublin university say that vitamin B12 appears to be an independent factor: in their study, women with the lowest as compared with the highest intakes of this nutrient were five times more likely to experience birth defects.

There have been claims that very large doses of vitamin B12 may reduce fatigue and improve mental function in the elderly, but there is little hard evidence to support this.

WHERE IS IT FOUND?

Huge amounts of vitamin B12 are found in liver and other organ meat. Eggs, milk, meat and fish supply lesser but adequate amounts. The vitamin is also found in seaweed and fortified foods.

vegans can fall short of the vitamin unless they eat plenty of fortified foods or seaweed

ARE YOU GETTING ENOUGH?

The RDA of vitamin B12 can be supplied by less than a teaspoon of liver OR 20 g salmon, OR 300 ml milk OR 40 g Start cereal. Anyone who includes animal products in their diet is likely to be receiving more than enough vitamin B12, but vegans can fall short of the vitamin unless they eat plenty of fortified foods or seaweed which is also a varying but rich source of the nutrient. Requirements are increased during breastfeeding, and some studies suggest that pregnant women and the elderly may also need more and could benefit from a supplement.

Serious deficiency of vitamin B12 can occur regardless of diet in people who are not producing enough intrinsic factor required for absorption. The result is pernicious anaemia, which must be treated with vitamin B12 injections. Pernicious anaemia often runs in families, resulting from a genetically determined abnormal immune response which destroys the mechanism for making intrinsic factor. The disease results in irregular red blood cells and tiredness but, in the longer term, serious neurological symptoms can develop, which are irreversible if not treated in time.

PLAYING SAFE

Extremely high intakes (even up to 3000 μg per day) of vitamin B12 are believed to be perfectly safe, but are not normally necessary in healthy people.

FOLIC ACID

Folic acid (also known as folacin and folate) is a B vitamin which has found fame for its many valuable uses in recent years. The RDA is 200 μg.

WHAT DOES IT DO?

Folic acid is needed for the vital process of cell division, and along with vitamin B12 aids the production of healthy red blood cells. It is also crucial for the development of an unborn baby –

> *Folic acid is crucial for the development of an unborn baby*

especially of the foetal spinal cord. It has now been proven that supplementing with folic acid during pregnancy can markedly decrease the risk of spina bifida.

Recent research shows that folic acid may also be able to reduce the risk of heart attack, especially amongst a significant proportion of middle-aged men who have a genetic abnormality in folic-acid metabolism. It does this by reducing levels of an amino acid called homocysteine.

There is some evidence that folic acid may help prevent precancerous cell changes. Low folic-acid levels are associated with early stage abnormalities in the cervix, colon and lung.

WHERE IS IT FOUND?
Good sources of folic acid include liver, pulses, vegetables (especially Brussels sprouts, potatoes, broccoli and spinach), oranges and fortified foods.

ARE YOU GETTING ENOUGH?
Consuming 90 g liver, OR 2–3 baked potatoes, OR 180 g boiled Brussels sprouts, OR 220 g boiled spinach, OR 80 g cornflakes will provide the RDA of folic acid. However this is not enough for pregnant women who require a daily 400 μg supplement in addition to the folic acid obtained through dietary means. For maximum protection, folic acid should be taken from prior to conception until the end of the twelfth week of pregnancy.

You may also be getting too little folic acid if you miss out on green leafy vegetables. Particularly at risk could be middle-aged males, the elderly and women taking the contraceptive pill.

PLAYING SAFE
Supplements are safe when taken as directed (up to 400 μg or 700 μg in the short term). However don't overdose because lots of folic acid can mask the serious neurological symptoms of a vitamin B12 deficiency. Excessive amounts can also deplete zinc and may interfere with epilepsy medication. Tell your doctor if you are taking folic acid.

BIOTIN

Biotin is the eighth and final water-soluble B vitamin. In some literature you might see it referred to by its old name – vitamin H. The RDA for biotin is 0.15 mg.

WHAT DOES IT DO?

Like many of the other B vitamins, biotin is involved in the metabolism of food components. It is of central importance in metabolising fats and helps in making a supply of essential glucose when energy intakes are low. Biotin is also known to be important in maintaining healthy skin and hair. However reports that it can treat hair loss and skin conditions are unfounded.

WHERE IS IT FOUND?

Small amounts of biotin are found in a wide variety of foods. The richest sources are organ meats and peanuts. Eggs, soya beans, fish, meat, wholemeal bread and cheese are also good sources, but fruit and vegetables contain very little.

> *Biotin is important in maintaining healthy skin and hair*

ARE YOU GETTING ENOUGH?

The RDA of biotin is supplied by 75 g chicken livers, OR 150 g peanuts, OR 19 boiled eggs OR 600 g cooked soya beans, OR 1.3 kg pilchards OR 2 kg Camembert cheese. Although the average intake of biotin (around 30 μg per day) is far lower than the EU RDA, other estimates of the requirement for biotin are much lower and deficiency is unknown in healthy adults eating a normal diet. However a scaly skin condition can be induced by the bizarre (and unhealthy) consumption of large amounts of raw egg whites which contain a factor that binds biotin. Biotin deficiency is more common in infants, but supplements of the vitamin should not be given to infants without medical advice.

PLAYING SAFE

There are no reported adverse effects from using biotin. The

Upper Safe Level for supplementation has been set at 2.3 mg per day.

VITAMIN C

Vitamin C – also known as ascorbic acid – is an important water-soluble nutrient which improves resistance to infection and helps maintain the health of our body cells and blood vessels. The RDA is 60 mg.

WHAT DOES IT DO?

Vitamin C is essential for the action of white blood cells which are the part of our immune defence system that scavenges bacteria and viruses. Whether vitamin C helps stave off colds has been a matter of great debate and disagreement over the years. The consensus now seems to be that vitamin C can definitely reduce the duration of a cold, although it isn't likely to impact on the actual number we catch. The *Scandinavian Journal of Infectious Diseases* (1994) carried a review of twenty studies where at least 1000 mg vitamin C was tested for its effects; although only some of the studies found a link with fewer colds, all of them reported milder symptoms. These results may be of practical significance in terms of fewer sick days lost from work or school.

Vitamin C is an important antioxidant which means it helps to protect body cells from attack by free radicals – highly reactive molecules that have been associated with diseases like cancer and heart disease. In particular, vitamin C is thought to help prevent cholesterol from becoming oxidised (rancid) – a phenomenon understood to be the precursor to 'furring' of arteries. In the stomach, vitamin C also prevents carcinogenic substances called nitrosamines being formed from nitrates in food.

Additionally, vitamin C is an important factor in healthy skin and gums. It promotes wound healing and is required for the formation of collagen – the 'cement' that holds our cells and tissues together and makes up the structure of blood vessels and capillaries.

Another important role for vitamin C is in improving iron absorption from plant-based foods. These sources of iron are much more poorly absorbed than meat sources, but eating them with vitamin-C rich foods can markedly improve the uptake of iron.

WHERE IS IT FOUND?
Virtually all fruits and vegetables (including potatoes) supply vitamin C. Oranges and other citrus fruits are often thought of as the best sources, but in fact blackcurrants and green peppers provide a richer supply.

ARE YOU GETTING ENOUGH?
It is easy to obtain the RDA of 60 mg vitamin C from a healthy diet: just 50 g green pepper, OR 150 ml orange juice, OR 2 small kiwis provides this amount. However, there is now increasing evidence that an optimum intake of vitamin C may be nearer 150 or 200 mg daily, and for a therapeutic effect in colds supplements of 1000 mg or more may be needed.

Smokers are most at risk of low vitamin C levels – the 1991 COMA (Committee on Medical Aspects of Food Policy) report on Dietary Reference Values suggests that the requirement for smokers could be up to 80 mg per day higher simply to keep vitamin C levels the same as in non-smokers.

fruit and vegetables (including potatoes) supply vitamin C

Severe deficiency of vitamin C leads to scurvy – now thankfully rare in the UK. Symptoms include bleeding gums, easy bruising and poor wound healing.

PLAYING SAFE
Based on extensive safety data, a sensible maximum daily intake of vitamin C is 2000 mg for most people. More than this may cause temporary diarrhoea. High intakes are not advisable for those with pre-existing kidney disease, but it is a myth that vitamin C initiates kidney stones in healthy people.

Some researchers have raised concern that high levels of vitamin C may potentiate the effect of the contraceptive pill and effectively turn a low-dose pill into a higher-dose, and therefore more dangerous, one. However there is no evidence that this could occur at doses of less than 1000–2000 mg daily.

VITAMIN D

Unlike other vitamins, vitamin D can be manufactured by the body – it is formed by the action of sunlight on a cholesterol derivative in the skin. In fact vitamin D is technically classified as a hormone, because it is formed in one organ (the skin), yet acts on distant organs (the gut and bones). The RDA is 5 μg.

WHAT DOES IT DO?

Vitamin D is crucial for the regulation of the bone minerals, calcium and phosphorus. When blood calcium levels start to fall, vitamin D hormone is secreted into the circulation and the intestinal absorption of calcium and

vitamin D plays a vital role in preventing bone deficiency diseases

phosphorus is increased. At the same time, the bones release more of these minerals into the blood stream, and the kidneys minimise the amount of calcium lost via the urine. The effect is the normalising of blood calcium levels which must be kept constant for correct nerve and muscle function.

Because vitamin D dramatically improves the absorption of calcium from food, the mineral plays a vital role in preventing bone deficiency diseases like osteoporosis in adults and rickets in children. Several studies have shown that a daily supplement of vitamin D reduces the risk of hip fractures in the elderly, and there is evidence that the vitamin can also reduce some of the pain and stiffness associated with osteoarthritis.

Recent studies also suggest that vitamin D influences cell division and could play a role in cancer development. In one scientific study, some breast cancer patients treated with surgery and radiation received follow-up vitamin D treatment and some didn't. In the group that received the treatment, seventy per cent remained healthy for a long period, whereas sixty per cent in the group who didn't receive vitamin D suffered a recurrence of their disease.

WHERE IS IT FOUND?

Good food sources of vitamin D are few and far between. The best sources are cod liver oil and halibut liver oil supplements. Liver, oily fish and tinned fish eaten with bones also provide good amounts; whilst full-fat dairy products, margarine and eggs contain much lesser amounts.

ARE YOU GETTING ENOUGH?

The RDA of vitamin D (5 μg) can be obtained from approximately 1 teaspoon cod liver oil, OR 20 g baked kipper or grilled herring, OR 67 g canned sardines, OR 100 g canned tuna, OR 5 eggs, OR 200 g butter, OR 14 l whole milk. Children and people over fifty need around double the RDA, whilst young adults who are healthy and spend some time outdoors can usually manufacture enough vitamin D to make a dietary source unnecessary. Exceptions include people with dark skin (which doesn't synthesise vitamin D very efficiently), breastfeeding women and those whose religious beliefs require them to keep their skin covered.

Elderly people, especially the housebound, are most likely to have the lowest levels of vitamin D and can suffer bone-deficiency problems as a result. Nearly all elderly people could benefit from taking a vitamin D supplement.

PLAYING SAFE

Fat-soluble vitamin D is stored in the body, so too much can build up and be harmful. Prolonged intakes of more than about 50 μg (2000 IU) can initiate symptoms of weight loss, poor appetite, nausea and depression. To allow a high margin of safety, it's recommended that the maximum daily intake from supplements should not exceed 10 μg (400 IU). However shorter-term intakes of up to 50 μg are perfectly acceptable and may be professionally recommended in certain cases.

VITAMIN E (TOCOPHEROL)

Vitamin E was originally identified as a fertility factor in rats, leading to wild claims that it was an aphrodisiac and cure for reproductive problems. Although these claims haven't turned out to be true, the vitamin is nonetheless vitally important for health, and new discoveries are being made about its benefits all the time. The RDA for the vitamin is 10 mg.

WHAT DOES IT DO?

Vitamin E is an important antioxidant nutrient – it helps stop fatty cell membranes becoming oxidised (rancid) and appears to play a role in protecting against free-radical mediated diseases such as cancer and heart disease. The vitamin is also needed for healthy red blood cells and proper functioning of the immune system.

An increasing amount of research shows that doses of vitamin E in excess of the basic RDA can help prevent or treat certain diseases. For example intakes of 300–400 mg daily have been found to improve symptoms of intermittent claudication (pain in the legs whilst walking, due to poor circulation). Similar amounts have also been shown to ease symptoms of premenstrual syndrome, and 200–800IU (134–156 mg) has been shown to normalise reduced immune function in older people.

Several studies have shown a promising effect of vitamin E in heart disease. In fact the results from a World Health Organisation trial indicate that vitamin E status is an even more important predictor of heart disease than blood pressure or blood cholesterol. In 1993, two large US studies involving male and female doctors and nurses found that heart attack risk was significantly reduced in those who took vitamin E supplements containing at least 100 IU (67 mg) daily. The strongest benefit came from regular use over two years.

Vitamin E helps improve dry skin

In 1995 a more tightly controlled study at the University of Cambridge also found a benefit of vitamin E in preventing heart attacks. Men already suffering from symptoms of heart disease, such as angina, were given 268–536 mg of the vitamin daily or a placebo. In the vitamin E supplemented group, there was a seventy-five per cent decrease in non-fatal heart attack compared with the placebo group.

Vitamin E is also commonly used as a constituent of beauty creams. It helps improve dry skin and may also protect against wrinkles and sun-ageing.

WHERE IS IT FOUND?

The only really significant source of vitamin E is wheat germ and wheat-germ oil. However other vegetable oils, especially sunflower oil, also contain reasonable amounts, as do nuts, avocados and sweet potatoes. Blackberries, tomatoes and chickpeas also contain some vitamin E, and other vegetables and meat sources contain traces.

ARE YOU GETTING ENOUGH?

The RDA of vitamin E can be obtained from 2–3 teaspoons wheat germ oil, OR approx 2 tablespoons sunflower oil, OR 45 g wheat germ, OR 40 g almonds, OR 2 medium avocados, OR 220 g sweet potato, OR 10 medium tomatoes, OR 420 g blackberries.

According to the *Nutritional and Dietary Survey of British Adults* (HMSO, 1990), the average daily intake of vitamin E from food is 9.9 mg in men and 7.2 mg in women – in both cases below the RDA. In one sense, this doesn't seem to be a problem, because there is no specific deficiency disease associated with taking low amounts. However, as we have seen, the intake for optimum health in the longer term may in fact be well above the RDA.

People most likely to benefit from taking a supplement of vitamin E include those at high risk of heart disease or cancer, people with circulation problems and people under stress (stress increases oxidation processes in the body). Pregnant and breastfeeding women also need more vitamin E, and the requirement for vitamin E is further increased by a high intake of polyunsaturated fats. These fats – found mostly in vegetable oils, nuts, seeds and oily fish – are thought to be more 'healthy' than the saturated kind, but they can easily become oxidised in the body, and extra vitamin E is needed to protect against this.

PLAYING SAFE

Vitamin E is the safest of the fat-soluble vitamins. Up to 800 mg daily as a supplement is considered harmless, but higher amounts may potentiate the effect of blood-thinning drugs (e.g. warfarin), or cause occasional gastrointestinal disturbance.

WHAT ARE FREE RADICALS AND ANTIOXIDANTS?

In the time it takes you to read this page, your body has taken trillions of hits from molecules called free radicals. Free radicals are a natural by-product of the process whereby food is made into energy, but they can also arise from outside sources like cigarette smoke, radiation and pollution. In excess, the molecules are potentially destructive because they have an unpaired electron (negative charge). In an attempt to become electrically balanced, they will strip electrons from any biological material, wreaking damage to important cellular structures and interfering with genetic material in the process.

The good news is that for the most part the body is very effective at using dietary antioxidants – in particular vitamin E, vitamin C, beta carotene and selenium – to neutralise excess free radicals and keep them from damaging body cells. But if the antioxidant status of the body falls low, through poor diet or free-radical overload, illness can result. Cancer, heart disease, cataracts and arthritis are all diseases believed to be related to free-radical activity in some way.

VITAMIN K

Vitamin K is an important fat-soluble vitamin that exists in two chemical forms: phylloquinones which are present in many vegetables, and menaquinones which are manufactured by bacteria. There is no EU RDA or British RNI for the vitamin, but the Committee on the Medical Aspects of Food Policy (COMA) has suggested that requirements are between 0.5 and 1 μg /kg body weight per day. In other words, a 70 kg person would require approximately 35–70 μg vitamin K daily.

WHAT DOES IT DO?
Vitamin K plays a crucial role in helping the blood to clot. Without vitamin K, the smallest cut could be devastating and could even result in haemorrhage.

WHERE IS IT FOUND?
All vegetables contain some vitamin K, but the best sources are green leafy varieties. Animal-based foods which naturally contain some bacteria, like milk, meat, cheese and butter, also contain a little vitamin K.

ARE YOU GETTING ENOUGH?
It is very rare under normal circumstances that adults fall short of vitamin K, and supplements are generally regarded as unnecessary. A study of ten male college students estimated that the intake of vitamin K from dietary sources was about 80 μg per day. The natural bacterial flora in the gut also produces a subsistence level of the vitamin regardless of intake from food.

Vitamin K plays a crucial role in helping the blood to clot

Adults who take blood-thinning drugs can, however, be at risk of vitamin K deficiency. Patients at risk may need to carry medically prescribed vitamin K ampoules, so that if they ever injure themselves, they can restore normal blood clotting as quickly as possible. Vitamin K deficiency can also be a serious problem in babies, and most newborns are also given vitamin K injections to prevent haemorrhaging.

PLAYING SAFE
Safety isn't really an issue, because vitamin K is so rarely available in supplements. However, according to COMA, natural vitamin K is remarkably free from side effects, even in milligram doses. Synthetic preparations (providing menadione) are more toxic and best avoided for nutritional purposes.

CHAPTER 4

Minerals

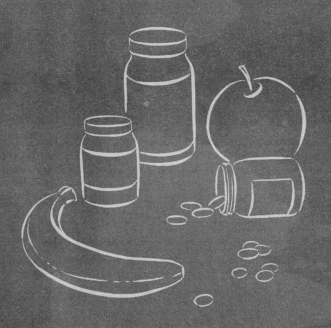

CALCIUM

Calcium is an important structural mineral, ninety-nine per cent of which is deposited in the skeleton. The RDA for the mineral is 800 mg, but a higher intake can be desirable for many population groups, especially women.

WHAT DOES IT DO?

Along with other minerals – in particular phosphorus and magnesium – calcium helps make bones and teeth dense and strong. Until the age of about thirty, it is possible to improve the density of the bones by laying down more calcium; hence a high consumption of the mineral in the early years is essential for preventing bone-deficiency diseases later in life.

Small amounts of calcium are also found in soft tissues and body fluids, and a constant concentration of calcium in the blood is essential for regulating nerve and muscle function. Vitamin D works with other hormones to regulate calcium

calcium helps make bones and teeth dense and strong

levels in blood and bone, and the vitamin is vital in promoting calcium absorption from the gut. This is why the two nutrients are often found together in supplements.

WHERE IS IT FOUND?

The very best sources of calcium are dairy products, with low-fat products being marginally richer in the mineral than the full-fat varieties. Calcium is also found in watercress, cabbage, broccoli and other greens, dried fruit (especially figs), pulses and oranges.

ARE YOU GETTING ENOUGH?

Despite the rich concentration of calcium in dairy products, you would still need to drink 680 ml skimmed milk a day or consume 90 g Cheddar cheese in order to obtain the entire RDA. If boiled broccoli was your only source of

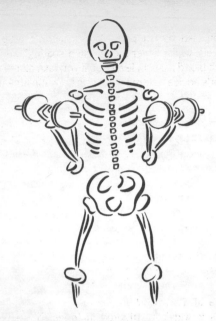

calcium, you would have to eat a massive 2 kg daily.

According to the *Dietary and Nutritional Survey of British Adults* (HMSO, 1990), the average intake of calcium by people in the UK reaches the RDA, but is below the levels of intake recommended by the National Osteoporosis Society. To minimise the chance of brittle bones, this charitable organisation recommends the following daily calcium intakes: 800 mg for children aged between seven and twelve; 1000 mg for teenagers, women up to forty-five, men up to sixty and women over forty-five on HRT; 1200 mg for pregnant and breastfeeding mothers; 1500 mg for pregnant and nursing teenagers, men over sixty and women over forty-five not on HRT.

PLAYING SAFE

Up to 1500 mg calcium daily is thought to be safe as a supplement, with any excess being easily excreted in the urine. Calcium kidney stones are usually only formed when the normal regulating mechanisms are no longer functioning, although lack of fluid can also play a part. Certain diuretic drugs reduce calcium levels, whilst other are 'calcium sparing', and actually increase the blood calcium level – so if you take diuretics, follow your doctor's advice before taking calcium supplements.

PHOSPHORUS

Phosphorus (phosphate) is an important part of all plant and animal cells. Over eighty per cent is found in the bones and teeth, and the RDA for the mineral is 800 mg.

WHAT DOES IT DO?
Phosphorus works alongside magnesium and calcium in building and maintaining healthy bones and teeth. The mineral is also vital for converting food into energy – it forms the 'phosphate' part of adenosine triphosphate (ATP) which is the basic unit of energy in every cell.

WHERE IS IT FOUND?
Phosphorus is widely distributed in foods, but especially in calcium-rich foods such as cheese, eggs, cream, skimmed-milk powder and in foods high in protein such as meat and poultry.

ARE YOU GETTING ENOUGH?
Surveys show that virtually everyone consumes well in excess of the RDA for phosphorus: just 400 g chicken OR 163 g Cheddar cheese will supply the daily amount, and there is some phosphorus in virtually every food. Interestingly it's estimated that on average, ten per cent of the daily requirement for phosphorus comes from additives, such as polyphosphates in meat and phosphoric acid in fizzy drinks.

in general, phosphorus intakes are too high

PLAYING SAFE
Because the body is efficient at getting rid of excess phosphorus, the mineral isn't toxic in high amounts. However, in general, phosphorus intakes are too high, and there is concern that

chronic consumption of amounts above the RDA can have a negative effect on calcium levels in the body. The upper safe limit for long-term consumption (from both food and supplements) is estimated to be 1500 mg a day.

ZINC

Zinc is an ingredient of items as diverse as nappy rash creams and rust-proofing paints, but it is also a vital mineral for our health too. The RDA for the mineral is 15 mg.

WHAT DOES IT DO?

Zinc is an antioxidant mineral needed for a healthy immune defence system, and for repair and renewal of skin cells. The mineral is important for reproductive health, and low zinc levels may result in reduced sperm count. Pregnant women with low blood levels of zinc also tend to give birth to smaller babies, and poor growth in the first few months of life has been associated with reduced levels of zinc in breast milk.

Zinc is important for reproductive health

Men have a high concentration of zinc in their prostate gland, and anecdotal reports indicate that benign enlargement of the prostate gland – causing increased frequency of urination in middle-aged men – can be improved by consuming extra zinc.

Zinc is also promoted as an aid to help with skin conditions such as acne or eczema. The theory behind zinc therapy lies in the fact that the mineral is necessary for normal cell division, tissue repair and renewal. Zinc is also necessary for the metabolism of fatty acids into important substances that help regulate our skin health.

Some clinical studies have also found that zinc (sucked as lozenges) helps nip cold symptoms in the bud, whilst others have shown no conclusive result. Whether or not zinc is effective may depend on the chemical form used and the dosage. Higher strengths of zinc gluconate appear to be the most effective.

WHERE IS IT FOUND?

The best sources of zinc include seafood, especially oysters (richer than any other food), lean beef, whole-grain cereals, sardines, liver and kidney, chickpeas and lentils. Milk and dairy products also contain some zinc.

enlargement of the prostate gland can be improved by consuming extra zinc

ARE YOU GETTING ENOUGH?

The RDA of zinc (15 mg) can be obtained from just 2–3 oysters, OR 300 g grilled rump steak, OR 450 g bran flakes, OR 15 slices wholemeal bread OR 650 g Cheddar cheese. The average daily intake of zinc actually achieved is around 11.4 mg for men and 8.4 mg for women. Although these intakes are below the EU RDA, they exceed the British RNIs (RNI for men = 9.5 mg, RNI for women = 7 mg).

Breastfeeding women and females in the 16–24 age group have increased requirements for zinc, and are amongst the groups most likely to be marginally deficient. Other groups affected include slimmers and pregnant women, as well as vegetarians and vegans. A diet extremely high in fibre can deplete zinc from the body and exacerbate a deficiency. Symptoms may include problems such as frequent infections, delayed wound healing, reduced appetite, decreased sense of taste and smell, poor skin condition and persistent white flecks on the nails (occasional white flecks are usually the result of a knock to the nail bed). There is also some evidence that low zinc levels are linked with aggressive and delinquent behaviour in young males.

Low zinc intakes may also affect fertility, and have been linked with the eating disorder anorexia nervosa. According to Professor Bryce-Smith, retired Professor of Organic Chemistry at Reading University, zinc deficiency may contribute to the anorexic condition by impairing the sense of taste and smell, and therefore the desire to eat.

PLAYING SAFE

Zinc is not in itself particularly unsafe, but there are concerns that high intakes can imbalance other minerals, such as iron and copper, in the body. For this reason, the maximum level allowed in supplements is 15 mg.

IRON

Iron is a vital trace mineral, needed only in small dietary amounts. The chemical symbol for iron is 'Fe', and on the labels of fortified foods and supplements, iron is often referred to as a 'ferrous' compound, such as ferrous sulphate.

The RDA for iron is 14 mg, although men are likely to need less than this, and women a little more. The British recommendation (RNI) for females between the ages of nineteen and fifty is 14.8 mg; this does not take into account the increased needs of women who lose a lot of blood through heavy monthly periods.

WHAT DOES IT DO?

Iron is a key part of haemoglobin – the pigment in red blood cells that transports oxygen from the lungs to other body tissues. We are most likely to become aware of iron's importance only when we fall short of the mineral: depletion of iron leads to iron-deficiency anaemia, a condition in which body tissues begin to 'suffocate' from lack of oxygen.

Depending on severity, iron deficiency can cause varying degrees of fatigue, dizziness, weakness, appetite loss, hair loss and lack of concentration. To prevent such symptoms, it is essential that iron intakes are kept adequate.

WHERE IS IT FOUND?

Iron is found in both animal- and plant-based foods, but animal sources are far better absorbed. This is because they provide 'haem' iron, the organic form of iron contained in our own blood. The best animal sources are cockles, mussels, liver, kidney, lean beef and other red meats, pilchards and sardines; the richest vegetable sources include fortified breakfast cereals, pulses (especially chickpeas), dried fruit (especially figs), avocados, nuts, deep green vegetables, whole-grain cereals and plain chocolate.

ARE YOU GETTING ENOUGH?

14.8 mg (the RNI) is the amount in 148 g fried lamb's liver, OR 123 g All Bran, OR 617 g plain chocolate, OR 987 g chickpeas, OR 1480 g broccoli. In practice vegetarians may need to eat a higher amount still, because of the relatively poor absorption from plant sources.

Iron-deficiency anaemia is the most common nutritional deficiency disease in the world. Overall it affects about ten per cent of women (mostly those with heavy periods or

iron will help prevent anaemia

who are pregnant), six per cent of post-menopausal women, and two per cent of men. Anaemia is usually diagnosed when haemoglobin levels fall, whereas a milder iron deficiency is marked by low iron stores without a significant reduction in haemoglobin.

Children are also likely to suffer iron deficiency, a phenomenon that has been linked with lower IQ. Women who have a low store at the beginning of pregnancy also risk becoming anaemic unless they are given supplements. You may also be at risk if you exercise heavily; in particular sustained movement in endurance sports like marathon running can break down red blood cells and cause tiny intestinal ruptures that lead to minor bleeding and iron loss.

If you suspect you are anaemic, get a blood test to confirm it. If the result is positive, chances are you will be prescribed much higher levels of iron than can normally be supplied by diet. It's important not to experiment with high-dose iron pills without medical advice, as excessive iron intake can be undesirable. However, taking a multivitamin that includes just the RDA of iron will help prevent anaemia and is probably desirable for many women.

PLAYING SAFE

For healthy individuals the maximum level of iron deemed safe for long time self-supplementation is 15 mg daily. If you don't need the extra iron, higher-dose supplements may prove harmful. This is because free iron accumulates in organs and tissues and may act as a catalyst to damaging oxidation reactions in the body.

One in 250 people carry a gene that leads to haemochromatosis, a condition that encourages the body to overload iron even if the person follows a normal diet. Symptoms include abdominal pain, bronzed skin, achy joints and an increased risk of cardiovascular disease. Sufferers should not take supplements of iron under any circumstances.

All iron supplements should be kept well out of the way of children, as accidental iron poisoning can be, and unfortunately often is, fatal.

IRON DEPLETERS AND ENHANCERS
There are various factors that improve or inhibit the uptake or non-haem iron from vegetable sources:

Enhancers include
Vitamin C (e.g. orange juice)
Fructose, sorbitol
Alcohol
Certain amino acids (in protein foods)

Depleters include
Tannins, polyphenols (tea, red wine)
Phosphates, phytates (high-fibre grains)
Bran
Egg protein, legume protein
Calcium

MAGNESIUM

Magnesium is a vital component of bones and teeth, and is sometimes known as the 'anti-stress' mineral because of its close connection with the nervous system.

WHAT DOES IT DO?

More than sixty-five per cent of the magnesium content of the human body is found in the bone where, along with calcium and phosphorus, it provides structure and strength.

Magnesium is needed for healthy nerves and muscles

Magnesium also plays a pivotal role in the release of energy from food, and is needed for healthy nerves and muscles. Magnesium supplements can be useful in women who suffer premenstrual symptoms such as cramps, sugar cravings and feeling blue. A lack of the mineral may lead to increased irritability, anxiety or mild depression. Restless leg syndrome, muscle spasms and twitchy eyelids may also signify a marginal magnesium deficiency.

As magnesium is involved in the contraction of heart muscle, low levels can sometimes be associated with dangerous arrhythmias (irregular beats or palpitations). Heart attack victims may be treated with magnesium sulphate injections to aid recovery, but oral doses of magnesium do not have the same therapeutic effect. Nevertheless eating a diet rich in magnesium will play a part in keeping the heart healthy, and a recent study in the *British Journal of Nutrition* suggests that magnesium supplements may also be able to reduce blood pressure.

A small study reported in the *Lancet* in 1991 also found that magnesium seemed to reduce muscle pain and increase energy in ME sufferers, but this has not been confirmed.

WHERE IS IT FOUND?

Nuts, whole-grain cereals and pulses are amongst the best sources of magnesium, although the mineral can also be found in dairy products, meat and seafood, bananas and green vegetables.

ARE YOU GETTING ENOUGH?

The RDA of magnesium (300 mg) is supplied by 73 g Brazil nuts, OR 10 Shredded Wheat, OR 769 g Edam cheese, OR 882 g cooked spinach.

According to the *Dietary and Nutritional Survey of British Adults* (HMSO, 1990), women consume on average only 237 mg magnesium per day, which is less than the RDA. Slimmers, heavy drinkers and people taking diuretic drugs are amongst those most at risk of low levels, and most likely to require a magnesium supplement.

PLAYING SAFE

There is no evidence that magnesium is harmful in healthy people, and supplements providing 300–400 mg daily are thought to be safe. However very high doses of magnesium (Epsom) salts taken for their purgative action can interfere with the transmission of nerve impulses.

SELENIUM

Once only recognised as a toxin, the trace mineral selenium is now established as being essential to health – albeit in tiny quantities. At present, there is no EU RDA for selenium, but the British Reference Nutrient Intake (RNI) is 60 μg per day for adult females and 75 μg a day for adult males.

WHAT DOES IT DO?

Selenium forms part of an antioxidant enzyme which stops the fatty parts of our cells turning rancid and which helps prevent cholesterol from assuming its oxidised (artery-clogging) form. The mineral also helps strengthen the body's immune responses.

According to Dr Margaret Rayman, a Research Fellow at the University of Surrey, low levels of selenium could contribute to cardiovascular disease, joint problems, cancer and subfertility. In one British study, women who had low levels of selenium in their blood had increased risk of miscarriage. Sperm motility has also been improved in subfertile men by a selenium supplement, and a recent US study showed 200 μg of selenium given daily reduced deaths from cancer by fifty per cent.

It's a popular belief that selenium supplements can also ease the pain and misery of arthritis, and several anecdotal reports back this up. Selenium helps facilitate production of anti-inflammatory chemicals in the body and although a definitive role in the disease remains unproven, levels have been reported to be depressed in rheumatoid-arthritis sufferers. In one report, published

> *Selenium helps strengthen the body's immune responses*

in the British Journal of Rheumatology in1992, there was a moderate benefit on pain and stiffness symptoms in sufferers who took 200 μg selenium per day.

The mineral is also required for the production of thyroxine, a hormone made by the thyroid gland which helps regulate metabolic rate.

Many selenium functions are closely linked with vitamin E, and the two have a synergistic (complementary) relationship.

WHERE IS IT FOUND?
Selenium is found in sources such as liver and kidney, fish, bread and other wheat-containing foods. Brazil nuts are the star source.

ARE YOU GETTING ENOUGH?
The RNI of selenium for adult females (60 μg) can be found in just a couple of Brazil nuts, OR 65 g lamb's kidney, OR 160 g steamed plaice. Old analyses of wholemeal bread indicate that 4–5 slices would also provide this amount, but in recent years levels have fallen in wheat flour. In fact, according to research at the Scottish Agricultural College in Ayr, dietary selenium intakes have dropped dramatically in Europe over recent years due to a switch from high-selenium Canadian wheat to a low-selenium locally grown variety. The current estimated intake is only 30–35 μg daily: when selenium intakes dropped this low in Finland, it was regarded as a national health hazard and the incorporation of selenium into fertilisers was made mandatory.

Those most prone to a deficiency of selenium include the elderly, pregnant and nursing mothers, people with arthritis, smokers and those with a generally poor diet. People who choose to supplement with selenium should take vitamins C and E. For good absorption, the selenium should also be in an 'organic' form, e.g. selenium yeast, amino acid chelated selenium or seleno-methionine.

PLAYING SAFE

Taking supplements of selenium up to 200 μg on a daily basis is considered quite safe for adults. But intakes of five times this amount are toxic, and may lead to nausea, nail loss, diarrhoea and garlic breath.

CHROMIUM

Chromium may be better known for its use in plating metals, but it is also an essential mineral in the diet. No EU RDA or British RNI has been set for the mineral, but it is thought that above 20 μg daily is not likely to cause any major deficiency symptoms. The Americans have set a 'safe and adequate' level for chromium intake of between 50 and 200 μg a day.

WHAT DOES IT DO?

Chromium is needed for the formation of a substance called glucose tolerance factor (GTF) which helps insulin in its job of regulating blood-sugar levels. A deficiency of chromium is associated with blood-sugar irregularities, and supplementing with the mineral has been reported to ease sugar cravings. Severe chromium deficiency is known to result in poor glucose tolerance, the precursor to diabetic conditions. A highly refined diet, with a large intake of sugars that require chromium for metabolism, could predispose some individuals to a chromium deficiency and aggravate adult-onset diabetes.

Some studies have also suggested that chromium supplements can be taken by athletes to enhance muscle development and discourage the laying down of fat. This is on the basis that chromium aids insulin function, which in turn encourages the uptake of amino acids (protein) into muscle. However its effectiveness as a sports supplement has yet to be fully proven, and there is no evidence that chromium can aid slimming.

Chromium is also purported to play a role in maintaining a

healthy, low cholesterol level. When glucose tolerance is impaired – a possible consequence of chromium deficiency – the liver manufactures more cholesterol; so maintaining an adequate intake of chromium could be important for a healthy heart.

WHERE IS IT FOUND?
Detailed analysis of the chromium contents of foods has not been carried out, but some of the best sources of chromium are believed to include whole grains, brewer's yeast, hard water, meat, kidneys and cheese.

ARE YOU GETTING ENOUGH?
According to the Committee on Medical Aspects of Food Policy, the average UK diet provides between 13.6 and 47.7 μg chromium daily, and some people at the lower end of this scale may be marginally deficient. For people wanting to safeguard their intake, chromium is present in some of the more comprehensive multivitamin and mineral formulations. Individual chromium supplements also exist at strengths of up to 100 or 200 μg. Chromium polynicotinate is thought to be particularly well absorbed as it mimics how the mineral occurs naturally in the GTF complex.

PLAYING SAFE
Chromium can be highly toxic in the 'hexavalent' chemical form, but the 'trivalent' form – found in food and supplements – has not been reported to cause harm. Supplements containing up to 200 μg are considered safe. However, if you are an insulin-dependent diabetic, it is best to take medical advice before taking chromium.

POTASSIUM

Potassium is one of four macrominerals and in fact is needed in higher amounts than any other mineral. There is no EU RDA, but the British RNI is set at 3500 mg a day for adult men and women.

WHAT DOES IT DO?

Potassium plays a fundamental role in maintaining the fluid and acid–alkaline balance of the body. It is vital for the transmission of nerve impulses, and is involved in helping the heart to beat regularly. Potassium also counterbalances sodium in the body, and is known to help lower blood pressure.

WHERE IS IT FOUND?

The best sources of potassium are fruit and vegetables, because they also provide a low level of sodium. However several other foods provide potassium, including wholemeal bread and pasta, brown rice, milk, fish and meat.

ARE YOU GETTING ENOUGH?

The RNI for potassium is supplied by 9 bananas, OR 14–15 oranges, OR 2.2 kg onions, OR 42 slices wholemeal bread.

The *Dietary and Nutritional Survey of British Adults* (HMSO, 1990) shows that the average intake of potassium is 3187 mg in males and 2434 mg in females. Compared with the RNI (3500 mg), intakes are low.

Potassium is vital for the transmission of nerve impulses, and is involved in helping the heart to beat regularly

Severe lack of potassium is rare, except in cases of acute diarrhoea or blood loss. Symptoms include mental confusion, listlessness, muscle weakness, irregular heart beat and respiratory failure.

People most at risk of marginal potassium include the elderly, athletes and manual workers who sweat a great deal and people taking certain diuretic drugs. There's also evidence that heavy coffee and alcohol drinkers may lack the mineral.

Most over-the-counter potassium supplements don't provide enough potassium for those people who have a medically induced need for the nutrient. But good multivitamins provide small amounts of the mineral, which help make up any marginal deficiency. The best way to achieve a sufficient intake of this mineral is to step up the intake of fruit and vegetables.

PLAYING SAFE
People with impaired heart or kidney function shouldn't take high-dose potassium supplements. Otherwise the mineral is quite safe, and acute toxicity has only been associated with doses above approximately 17 g a day – virtually impossible to achieve through oral intakes.

MANGANESE

Manganese has only fairly recently been recognised as an essential mineral for humans. There is no EU RDA or British RNI for the mineral, but safe intakes are estimated to lie above 1.4 mg a day for adults.

WHAT DOES IT DO?
Manganese aids in the development and maintenance of healthy bones and in the synthesis of substances called mucopolysaccharides that surround and lubricate the joints. The mineral is also required for sex hormone synthesis and is involved in antioxidant activity within the body.

WHERE IS IT FOUND?
Tea is estimated to provide half the amount of manganese in the British diet. Whole grains, nuts and avocados are rich sources, with other fruits and vegetables also containing moderate amounts.

ARE YOU GETTING ENOUGH?
The minimum daily intake thought to be adequate (1.4 mg) is supplied by 5 mugs of tea, OR 4.5 avocados, OR 70 g roasted peanuts. Manganese intakes have been estimated at around 4.6 mg per day so there is little evidence of deficiency in most individuals.

PLAYING SAFE

In long-term trials, manganese supplements have been found to be safe up to 15 mg daily.

IODINE

Iodine is an essential trace mineral. The EU RDA is 150 µg.

WHAT DOES IT DO?

Iodine is essential for the formation of thyroid hormones which regulate the body's metabolic rate. Through its effect on the thyroid, the mineral controls the production of energy, promotes growth and development, and helps burn fat.

WHERE IS IT FOUND?

The best dietary sources of iodine are fish and seafood. However bread and dairy foods are the main sources in the British diet.

ARE YOU GETTING ENOUGH?

The RDA for iodine can be found in 650 g mussels (weighed with shells), OR 60 g steamed haddock, OR 254 g canned salmon, OR 1 l milk. Iodine deficiency was once fairly widespread in England, and can still occur in certain communities. Particular areas, such as Derbyshire, have very little

> Iodine regulates the body's metabolic rate

iodine in the soil which means that locally grown foods are very low in the nutrient. Symptoms of iodine deficiency include tiredness, physical and mental slowness, weight gain, facial puffiness and constipation. Babies born to iodine-deficient mothers are lethargic and difficult to feed. Left untreated they develop cretinism with poor growth and mental retardation.

Most at risk of iodine deficiency are people such as strict vegetarians who eat no seafood or dairy products. Excessive intake of raw cabbage or nuts can also reduce the uptake of iodine into the thyroid gland and lead to deficiency.

If you feel you may be at risk of iodine deficiency, the best way to increase your intake is to use iodised salt (available from supermarkets and health food stores) or to take a kelp supplement. Kelp is a seaweed that is extremely rich in iodine.

> *Babies born to iodine-deficient mothers are lethargic and difficult to feed*

PLAYING SAFE

Large doses of iodine can be toxic. If you are taking it as a supplement it is important to read labels carefully and not take more than 500 μg per day (700 μg per day is acceptable for a month or so). Excess can lead to fast heart beat, anxiety, blurred vision and vomiting.

COPPER

Copper is an essential trace mineral. There is no EU RDA for copper, but the British RNI is 1.2 mg.

WHAT DOES IT DO?

Copper plays an important role in the development of red blood cells, and in the pigmentation that colours hair and skin. It also helps the body use vitamin C, and is essential for the formation of collagen and elastin – connective proteins found in ligaments, blood-vessel walls and the lungs. In addition, copper is a vital factor for strong bones and is also required for central nervous system activity.

Copper has been claimed to be useful in reducing cholesterol levels; however studies on humans have been inconsistent. Similarly any value of copper in psoriasis and rheumatoid arthritis has not been proved.

WHERE IS IT FOUND?

Most unprocessed foods contain some copper. Liver, shellfish, nuts, mushrooms, whole-wheat cereals and pulses (not canned) are good sources. Soft water may also dissolve copper in copper pipes.

ARE YOU GETTING ENOUGH?

The RNI for copper can be found in 11 g calf's liver, OR 70 g lobster, OR 120 g almonds, OR 167 g mushrooms, OR 12–13 slices wholemeal bread. The Dietary and Nutritional Survey of British Adults (HMSO, 1990) showed the average intake of copper was 1.6 mg per day in men and 1.2 mg per day in women – i.e. equal to or above the RNI. Severe copper deficiency is rare and people eating normal, unrestricted diets don't need to worry about their intake. However breastfeeding women, who have higher requirements, and people with a poor diet can safeguard their intake by taking a multivitamin and mineral supplement that contains copper. Symptoms of deficiency include anaemia and bone abnormalities.

PLAYING SAFE

Very high levels of copper can be toxic, producing destruction of red blood cells and liver and kidney damage. High doses of copper also reduce zinc absorption. These intakes are extremely unlikely from supplements, as the maximum level allowed in supplements is 5 mg.

OTHER TRACE MINERALS

Boron
Functions Studies indicate that boron can affect the composition, structure and strength of bone. Supplements may reduce bone loss in women after the menopause.
Sources Vegetables, nuts, dried fruit, wine, beer and honey contain boron. Dairy products, fish and meat also supply small amounts of the mineral.
Requirements The estimated requirement is around 2 mg per day.
Deficiency No precise signs and symptoms of boron deficiency have been defined.

Molybdenum
Functions Needed for iron metabolism and in the production of uric acid (a waste product found in blood and urine). Also

needed for normal sexual functioning in males.

Sources Relatively widespread in food.

Requirements The estimated safe intake is 50–400 μg daily.

Deficiency Deficiency is uncommon and there is no known deficiency disease.

Silicon

Functions Plays an important role in the manufacture of bone, cartilage and collagen.

Sources Whole-grain cereals and root vegetables are the best sources.

Requirements Requirements are estimated at 5–20 mg a day.

Deficiency The extent of deficiency is unknown but may contribute to bone weakness and skin and nail ailments.

Nickel

Functions The exact biochemical functions of nickel in the human body are unknown.

Sources Tiny amounts are found in a variety of food sources.

Requirements The requirement is not known, but current daily intakes – which appear to be adequate – are between 140 and 150 μg per day.

Deficiency In animals, deficiency leads to depressed growth and blood disorders.

Sodium

Functions Vital for maintaining the fluid and acid–alkaline balance of the body. Also closely involved in the function of nerves and muscles.

Sources Mainly salt (sodium chloride), but some foods also contain small amounts of naturally occurring sodium.

Requirements The Reference Nutrient Intake (RNI) is 1600 mg.

Deficiency Deficiency is very rare: high intakes are much more common and may lead, in sensitive individuals, to high blood pressure.

Chloride

Functions Chloride (negative) acts as the electrical counterbalance to sodium and potassium (positive) in the body's cells and tissues.

Sources The main source is salt (sodium chloride).

Requirements The Reference Nutrient Intake (RNI) is 2500 mg.

Deficiency Deficiency is very rare. Most people ingest more than enough chloride, and it may join sodium in contributing to raised blood pressure.

Sulphur

Function Needed to form keratin, a protein found in our hair and nails.

Sources Shellfish, beef, eggs, chicken, pork and pulses contain sulphur, as do all high-protein foods.

Requirements There is no official RDA or RNI for sulphur, and our exact needs are unknown.

Deficiency Deficiency is very unlikely with normal diets. The body gets all the sulphur it needs from high-protein foods, and doesn't require a separate dietary source.

CHAPTER 5

Other common supplements

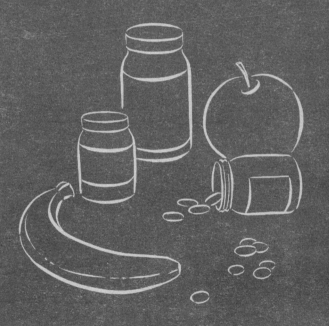

Walk into any health-food or drug store and, as well as vitamins and minerals, you'll find a wealth of other supplements lining the shelves, including oils, herbs, energy boosters and pick-me-ups. But do you really need any of these supplements, and if so how could they benefit your health? This chapter investigates some of the more common products available.

FISH OIL

Fish oil is a term encompassing liver oils (obtained from the liver of white fish such as cod and halibut) and fish-oil concentrate (obtained from the flesh of oily fish such as salmon). Cod liver oil supplements are rich in vitamins A and D, and contain variable amounts of the omega 3 polyunsaturates, eicosapentaenoic acid (EPA) and docosahexaenoic acid (DHA); supplements of fish oil concentrate are rich in EPA and DHA but do not contain vitamins A or D.

EPA is an active ingredient of fish oil involved in producing important hormone-like substances called prostaglandins. The prostaglandins produced from EPA help to:

- Reduce the stickiness of the blood, making it less liable to clot and cause thrombosis.
- Reduce levels of 'triglyceride' blood fats.
- Modestly reduce blood pressure.

These combined effects, together with a low-fat diet and healthy lifestyle, could result in a reduced risk of cardiovascular disease. In one study published in the Lancet, two to three fish meals a week, or an equivalent intake of fish oil, significantly reduced mortality in men who had already had one heart attack.

Some of the prostaglandins made from EPA are also anti-inflammatory. EPA-rich fish oils may therefore help relieve conditions such as psoriasis and arthritis in which inflammation is an important factor.

The DHA in fish oils – and also in breast milk – is an essential component of brain and eye tissue. Research shows that a rich intake of DHA is vital to brain development in infants. Failure to accumulate sufficient DHA has been shown to impair a child's learning ability, so pregnant and breastfeeding mothers should try to ensure a good intake of oily fish (or take fish oil capsules). For vegetarians, DHA can be made in

two to three fish meals a week significantly reduced mortality in men who had already had one heart attack

the body from linolenic acid – found in linseeds, rapeseed oil and green leafy vegetables.

Currently, our combined intake of EPA and DHA is only around 1 g per week, but the British Nutrition Foundation, in its 1993 briefing paper 'Nutritional Aspects of Fish', recommended that we should be consuming eight to ten times this – an amount roughly equivalent to at least 1–2 servings of fatty fish a week (mackerel, herring, salmon, pilchards, sardines), OR 1 teaspoon cod liver oil daily, OR 4 x 1 g fish oil concentrate capsules daily.

Before you choose a fish oil supplement, decide what you want from it. If you simply require the RDA of vitamins A and D to help maintain healthy bones, skin, mucous passages (e.g. respiratory tract) and immune system, the most basic cod liver oil or halibut liver oil capsules will do.

However, if you want fish oil to help maintain a healthy heart, or to ease the joints, look out for high quantities of EPA and DHA. As a rule, regular cod liver oil and halibut liver oil capsules only provide low levels of these fatty acids, high-strength cod liver oil capsules have low to medium levels, fish oil concentrate capsules provide medium levels and cod liver oil taken as a liquid supplies the highest amounts.

PLAYING SAFE

Cod liver oil contains vitamins A and D which in large excess can be toxic. So don't take more cod liver oil than recommended, and watch when you are combining it with other supplements that may provide vitamins A and D, particularly if you are pregnant. Very large amounts of EPA and DHA may thin the blood, so if you are taking anti-coagulant medication (e.g. warfarin or daily low-dose aspirin), take medical advice before taking anything other than regular amounts of fish oil.

Contrary to popular opinion, high-dose fish oil can also have the effect of actually increasing total cholesterol levels, especially in people eating a high-fat diet. However it increases the 'good' (HDL) type of cholesterol more than the 'bad' (LDL) type.

Fish oil contains highly polyunsaturated fatty acids which increase the need for the antioxidant vitamin E. If possible you should therefore take a product that is also fortified with this vitamin.

EVENING PRIMROSE OIL

Evening primrose oil has found fame as a supplement because it contains a very unusual fatty acid called gamma linolenic acid (GLA). There are no usual dietary sources of GLA, and under normal circumstances it is made in the body from the omega 6 polyunsaturate, linoleic acid – widely available in vegetable oils.

Some people have difficulty in this conversion process, and for them a direct source of GLA in the form of evening primrose oil is particularly beneficial. For example dyslexics, hyperactive children and people with eczema and asthma may not be able to make sufficient GLA. Stress, alcohol, saturated fats, ageing and vitamin or mineral deficiency (especial lack of zinc) can also affect GLA production.

GLA is also important because it is needed for the manufacture of particular prostaglandins (hormone-like substances) involved in regulating the immune system, circulation, skin and menstrual cycle.

Many women take evening primrose oil prior to menstruation to ease premenstrual symptoms. In one study, sixty-one per cent of PMS patients reported complete relief, and thirty-five per cent partial relief, whilst taking the oil. The best improvement appears to be in breast pain caused by benign cysts, and GLA is available on prescription to treat this condition. Evening primrose oil is also popular as a supplement during the menopause, although a study in the *British Medical Journal* found no significant benefit in the treatment of hot flushes.

> *take evening primrose oil prior to menstruation to ease premenstrual symptoms*

Evening primrose oil helps in maintaining good skin condition, partly by directly supplying fatty acids which help maintain skin cell membranes and 'lock in' moisture. Many women take evening primrose oil simply because they find it improves the smoothness of skin, enhances hair lustre and strengthens nails. The oil is also documented to help ease the more serious skin affliction, eczema. Some doctors actually prescribe GLA for this condition, but the level used has to be high and can be expensive. It's thought that evening primrose oil may help to dampen down the over-reaction of the immune system that can be at the root of atopic (allergic) conditions such as eczema.

In rheumatoid arthritis, where it's thought the body's own immune system begins attacking the joints, evening primrose oil may also be recommended. A study at Glasgow Royal Infirmary found that the oil helped sufferers reduce the amount of anti-inflammatory drugs they took, especially when taken in conjunction with fish oils.

Evening primrose oil is sometimes recommended in multiple sclerosis to correct a fatty-acid imbalance often seen in the disease; this usage should be discussed with your doctor.

Many people don't get results with evening primrose oil because they don't take enough. As a purely cosmetic supplement, 500–1000 mg is fine, but you'll need more if you have PMS, rheumatoid arthritis or eczema. In fact the minimum amount that seems to have any effect in these situations is around 2000 mg per day. You'll also need to persevere for at least three or four months.

If you are taking evening primrose oil it might also be advisable to take a multivitamin. This is because the efficacy of evening primrose oil depends on certain co-factor nutrients that process GLA into prostaglandins.

PLAYING SAFE

As with fish oils, evening primrose oil is very safe, but excessive levels may thin the blood, so never take more than the recommended dosage if you are using warfarin or a similar anticoagulant drug. Evening primrose oil should also be avoided by epileptics or schizophrenics, as it may interact with the drugs taken for these conditions.

Evening primrose oil contains highly polyunsaturated fatty acids which increase the need for the antioxidant vitamin E. If possible you should therefore take a product that is also fortified with this vitamin.

GARLIC

Garlic has been used as food and medicine throughout the ages. It was supposedly consumed by Egyptian pyramid builders for strength, and in the First World War was used as an antiseptic for soldiers' wounds. More recently, some of garlic's traditional uses have been borne out by scientific research.

Garlic has a long history as a natural remedy for colds and infections

The active components of garlic are believed to be sulphur compounds which have a beneficial effect on the immune system, heart and circulation. Garlic has a long history as a natural remedy for colds and infections, and as part of a healthy, low-fat diet, it can also have a beneficial effect on cholesterol levels, blood pressure and the 'sticki-

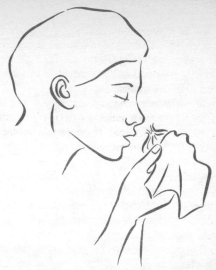

ness' of the blood. Certain compounds derived from garlic are also believed to act as antioxidants that protect cells and tissues from damage.

An intact garlic clove contains a sulphur compound called alliin, which is odourless. However, when a garlic clove is crushed, alliin comes into contact with an enzyme called alliinase, and the smelly anti-bacterial substance, allicin, is formed. Further conversion leads to a whole range of beneficial sulphur compounds being formed.

GARLIC SUPPLEMENTS EXPLAINED

Garlic oil capsules provide essential oil of garlic diluted in a base of vegetable oil. The essential oil is usually steamed or distilled from the garlic, and each clove only yields a tiny amount of concentrated oil. Hence garlic oil products only tend to be a few milligrams in strength, typically 0.66 mg, 2 mg or 4 mg per capsule.

Garlic oil products are most commonly used to provide some symptomatic relief in cases of colds and catarrh. About 4 mg garlic oil daily can also bring about some beneficial effects on the cardiovascular system.

Unfortunately, garlic oil, which mainly contains oily sulphides, is also a potent source of garlic odour. However, odour masking can be achieved by modifying the capsule shell, or by adding peppermint or parsley. Garlic oil may also be slightly irritant if you have a sensitive digestive system.

Powdered garlic products with an 'enteric' (protective) coating are designed to release allicin direct into the intestines. The cloves have to be sliced carefully and dried before being made into tablets, so that the alliinase enzyme is left unreacted. Allicin is then made in the body when the supplement reaches the intestines. It's important that the special 'enteric coat' is present as this lets aliinase, the enzyme needed to make allicin, escape from attack by stomach acid. It also means that any odour from the product is minimised.

A suitable dosage of allicin-releasing garlic tablets is around 600 mg a day, or as directed. This dosage can offer cardiovascular, anti-bacterial and other general garlic benefits.

Aged garlic extract contains mostly odourless water-soluble compounds and relatively smaller amounts of oil-soluble compounds. It is made by crushing fresh garlic and allowing it to 'age' in large tanks for around twenty months. During the ageing process, alliin and allicin are gradually 'bioconverted' into a range of other sulphur-containing compounds Aged garlic is available in tablet dosages from 100-600 mg. For daily 'maintenance', a lower level of 100–300 mg is sufficient; 1000 mg may be needed for more specific health benefits. Studies show that these levels may help reduce cholesterol levels and boost the immune system.

PLAYING SAFE

On the whole, garlic – whether eaten or used as a supplement – is fairly safe. Really huge levels can cause anaemia, and the raw herb should never be rubbed into the skin or used as a poultice as it can burn.

COENZYME Q10

Coenzyme Q10 (CoQ10) is a naturally occurring fat-soluble

substance found in every cell in the body. It is also known as a ubiquinone, from the Latin word meaning 'everywhere'.

People with low energy levels report great benefit from taking CoQ10

CoQ10 acts as an important coenzyme (facilitator) in the series of complicated chemical steps that release energy from food. The coenzyme can be made in the body but is also in rich supply in animal foods, such as organ meats, beef, sardines and mackerel. Peanuts and soya oil also contain relatively good amounts, but on the whole, people with solely vegetarian diets are less likely to receive a full complement of CoQ10 from food.

Nobody really knows how common low levels of CoQ10 are, but it is thought that ageing and illness can result in insufficient synthesis of the coenzyme with the result that levels decline. People with low energy levels associated with chronic fatigue illnesses often report great benefit from taking CoQ10, and the supplement benefits many older people and athletes too.

Certain heart conditions can also benefit from CoQ10, and the supplement has been shown to increase oxygen utilisation by the heart muscle. Research in the USA and in Japan has shown that hypertension (high blood pressure) can also respond in some cases to CoQ10.

Another area of interest is oral health, where a lack of CoQ10 may be associated with periodontal (gum) disease. A number of studies have shown that CoQ10 supplements can help diseased gums.

Supplements of CoQ10 come mainly in 10 mg, 15 mg and 30 mg strengths. A good starting level if you feel you may be low in CoQ10 is 15–30 mg daily. Signs may include unexplained tiredness (not related to lack of sleep or anaemia) and always feeling the cold. The elderly, vegetarians and vegans, and those who have been ill may be especially vulnerable to low levels of CoQ10.

PLAYING SAFE
CoQ10 seems to be a safe substance, and has been used

clinically at up to 150 mg daily without any toxicity problems. However very high doses may magnify the effect of anticoagulant (blood-thinning) drugs such as warfarin.

PROPOLIS

Bee propolis (or 'bee glue') is a sticky substance collected by bees from plants and trees. Together with beeswax, it is used to build the beehive. About half of bee propolis is resin, the rest is made up of wax, essential oils and pollen, plus trace amounts of vitamins, minerals and bioflavonoids.

Propolis has a natural antibiotic action, and may help the body's defences by neutralising foreign microbes. It also seems to have an anti-viral and anti-fungal action. The active agents are as yet not fully known, but antioxidant substances called bioflavonoids are thought to be one of the key ingredients.

Traditionally, propolis has been used for healing cuts, sores and wounds. It may also help combat sore throats and coughs. Other reported uses include helping to prevent peptic and duodenal ulcers, on the basis that propolis helps fights Helicobacter pylori, the bacterium involved in some ulcer conditions. However this use is unproven.

Propolis is available in capsules, as a tincture and in lozenges.

PLAYING SAFE
Propolis has a very good safety record and does not appear to have any side effects. A few years ago there were some problems with lead contamination of certain propolis samples, but this problem has now been resolved.

Propolis has a natural antibiotic action

ROYAL JELLY

This is a milky food produced by worker bees for the sustenance of their queen. Royal jelly has been heralded as a miracle cure, but health claims concerning the substance have been largely unsubstantiated. It contains only trace amounts of certain vitamins and other nutrients.

People take royal jelly as a 'pick-me-up'; and some claim that their hair, skin and nails improve with regular use. Fresh royal jelly capsules are the most popular, and purists argue that freeze-dried (or 'lyophilized') is not as good. Such claims are hard to prove.

> People take
> royal jelly as a
> 'pick-me-up'

PLAYING SAFE

Allergic reactions have very occasionally been reported in asthma sufferers taking royal jelly. However, in general, there are no problems associated with its use.

KELP

Kelp is a general name applied to various seaweed species. When eaten as a food, kelp provides large amounts of several minerals. However, in tablet form as a supplement, the only mineral it provides in significant amounts is iodine.

Because of its high iodine content, kelp can be taken to stimulate a slightly underactive thyroid gland (symptoms include sluggishness, fatigue, excess weight). However when comparing kelp products, the main points to look for are how much iodine you will get per daily dose (EU RDA = 150 μg), and how many tablets you need to take daily. Kelp is sometimes included in products aimed at slimmers, but it won't help weight loss if you are not deficient in iodine, and even then it is still necessary to follow a calorie-controlled diet.

> Kelp supplements
> should be avoided
> during pregnancy

PLAYING SAFE

Never take more than the stated dosage of kelp, as high levels of iodine can cause serious side effects. Kelp supplements should be avoided during pregnancy, or if you are taking medication for a thyroid problem.

SPIRULINA AND CHLORELLA

These are two types of freshwater micro-algae, with broadly similar nutritional profiles. Both may be consumed as a powdered food or as a supplement, but a typical intake from tablets (3 g a day) only provides nutritionally significant amounts of beta carotene, vitamin B12, iron and selenium. As foods (in amounts of around 20 g) spirulina and chlorella provide significant amounts of a much wider range of nutrients and are a source of high-quality plant protein. In addition, spirulina can be a good provider of the important fatty acid, GLA (100 mg per 10 g).

spirulina and chlorella are a source of high-quality plant protein

Spirulina, and especially chlorella, contain high concentrations of chlorophyll, the green plant pigment. In high levels, it is claimed that chlorophyll can help to remove heavy metals (lead, mercury, etc.) from the body, and to reduce the effects of radiation.

These 'green super foods' are becoming more popular with vegans and vegetarians, but when used as a supplement, a large number of tablets need to be taken to obtain a beneficial level of nutrients. However, fans claim that the enzymes and other 'whole food' factors found in spirulina and chlorella provide added benefits.

PLAYING SAFE

Spirulina and chlorella are not associated with any side effects as long as they are purchased from a reputable source and used according to the instructions.

ST JOHN'S WORT

St John's wort (also called Hypericum) is a herb that has proven benefits in relieving mild to moderate depression. It has been better researched than virtually any other herb and has fewer side effects than traditional anti-depressants.

St John's wort increases levels of a mood-lifting brain chemical called serotonin, and also elevates other important transmitters involved in combating depression. (There's evidence that the herb may also help with Seasonally Affective Depression, brought on by the short days of winter.)

> St John's wort is a herb that has proven benefits in relieving mild to moderate depression

Health professionals have been slow to latch on to St John's wort because it seems incredible that a humble herb could work so well to improve the mood. But in Germany the herbal extract is prescribed twenty times more commonly than any other anti-depressant. In 1994, a major psychiatric journal devoted an entire issue to the workings of the herb. St John's wort received a further credibility boost in 1996, when the prestigious British Medical Journal declared that the herb was 'significantly superior to placebo'.

A daily intake of St John's wort should provide around 900 μg of the active ingredient (hypericin) for best effect. It is recommended you take the herb for at least a month.

PLAYING SAFE
St John's Wort should not be taken by people who are more than moderately depressed and advice should be taken before taking the herb with other medications, especially anti-depressants.

GLUCOSAMINE

Glucosamine is an 'amino sugar' – a cross between a protein and a carbohydrate formed naturally in the body from glucose. Glucosamine is used in the manufacture of structural components such as connective tissue and collagen, and is vital for the formation of the cartilage and synovial fluids that help cushion the joints.

As the body ages, the ability to form glucosamine can decrease. Some scientists believe that deterioration of the joints with age – in particular osteoarthritis – may be worsened by inadequate glucosamine levels, and that taking a supplement could help. In one study on patients with osteoarthritis of the knee, the effects of a glucosamine supplement were compared with that of ibuprofen – a common painkiller and anti-inflammatory. After eight weeks, glucosamine emerged as the most favourable long-term treatment.

Glucosamine is also a popular supplement with athletes and sports people. It is usually found in the form of glucosamine sulphate in supplements (tablets or capsules). The recommended level of glucosamine sulphate intake is up to 1500 mg initially, and 500–1000 mg as a maintenance dose.

PLAYING SAFE
There are no known toxicity problems associated with taking glucosamine supplements.

GINSENG

Ginseng is made from the dried root of a herb called Panax, and has been used for many centuries in the East. A number of extravagant claims have been made for ginseng, including aphrodisiac and anti-ageing properties. It is also claimed to be an 'adaptogen' (something that restores harmony to body processes) and to aid vitality.

Several studies on animals have indicated that ginsenosides, the active ingredients of ginseng, do indeed have an effect in increasing adaptability to stress, increasing stamina, reducing blood pressure and inflammation and improving sleep. In humans, not all these benefits have been proved, but studies have shown an increase in stamina and concentration through taking the herb.

PLAYING SAFE
Ginseng is relatively non-toxic, but in high doses (above 3 g

daily) it has been linked with over-excitability, poor sleep and possible oestrogenic effects (e.g. breast tenderness in women). It should not be taken during pregnancy.

ECHINACEA

Echinacea is an important herb which has antiseptic and anti-viral properties and also helps dilate blood vessels. Traditionally it was used as a 'blood purifier' in the management of conditions such as boils and abscesses.

Echinacea is still sometimes used to relieve minor skin conditions, but more commonly it is taken to boost the immune system. It has been shown to stimulate white blood cell activity and to increase resistance to cold and flu viruses.

Echinacea is available as tincture or tablets and should be taken according to the instructions. Doses may be stepped up if you have an infection.

PLAYING SAFE
People taking immunosuppressant drugs should not take echinacea as it may interfere with these medications. There is also no safety data for use during pregnancy or breastfeeding, so it is probably best avoided at these times.

Echinacea is taken to boost the immune system

GINKGO BILOBA

Ginkgo biloba (Maidenhair) is a herbal preparation derived from the world's oldest tree. The active ingredients of ginkgo, called ginkgo flavonglycosides, are not found in any other plant species. They are known for their ability to improve circulation, particularly to the brain, hands and feet.

Ginkgo biloba can be of particular use for sufferers of cold hands and feet, or for those with intermittent claudication – a condition of poor circulation characterised by pain in the legs on walking. Supplements have also been shown to improve mental function, including confusion and poor memory in elderly people. But there is no evidence that they help boost mental capacity in younger people.

The effective daily dosage proven by clinical trials is 100–150 mg of a ginkgo extract which provides twenty-four per cent (24–36 mg) ginkgo flavonglycosides. Labels can be very confusing, so read carefully to avoid being misled!

> *Ginkgo biloba can be of particular use for sufferers of cold hands and feet*

PLAYING SAFE

Ginkgo biloba has few reported side effects at the dosages in normal use. However, people taking heart medications should take medical advice before using ginkgo. It may also be best to avoid the herb during pregnancy.

ALOE VERA

Aloe vera – also known as aloe barbadesis – has been valued for its medicinal uses for many years. The part of the plant used in most aloe vera products is the gel which lies deep within the leaves; the outer parts of the leaves contain a bitter laxative substance called aloin (hence 'bitter aloes'), which is discarded in manufacture.

More than ninety-eight per cent of aloe vera is water, but anti-inflammatory and antiseptic principles have also been identified in the gel, and soothing substances called mucopolysaccharides are believed to contribute to its beneficial qualities. Taken internally, aloe vera juice (processed directly from the gel) is reported to ease the discomfort of irritable bowel syndrome but there are no scientific studies to prove this.

A study published in the *Journal of Alternative Medicine* indicates that yeast infections can also be tackled with aloe vera. Yeast overgrowth in the stools was reduced in people who consistently took two teaspoons of aloe vera juice twice a day. The natural juice appears to have an anti-fungal action, as well as improving the overall balance of bacteria in the bowel.

Aloe vera is famed for its ability to heal skin conditions. Small open skin wounds treated with the gel have been shown to heal twice as fast as those left untreated, and the gel can also help sooth minor burns. A recent study has shown that topically applied aloe vera gel may be very effective at helping to clear psoriasis.

> *Aloe vera is famed for its ability to heal skin conditions*

PLAYING SAFE
There are no known side effects attributable to the normal use of aloe vera.

CHAPTER 6

Special vitamin needs

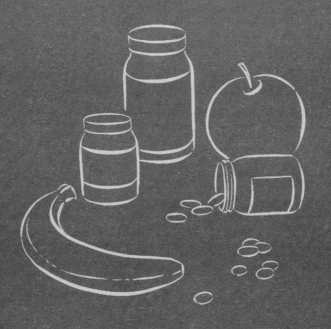

Particular lifestyles or life stages may mean an increased demand for certain nutrients. For example women have greater vitamin requirements during pregnancy and lactation, and young children and the elderly also have special nutritional needs. Similarly, highly active people have high energy requirements and need correspondingly more vitamins and minerals, while people who smoke rob their bodies of valuable antioxidants that need to be replaced. Vegetarians and vegans don't in themselves have higher nutrient needs, but may need to plan their diets more carefully to ensure they achieve an adequate vitamin intake.

UNDER FIVES

Emphasis on: vitamin D, iron
Healthy adults can manage without a source of vitamin D (the vitamin can be made through the action of sunlight on skin), but it's essential that the under fives get a dietary supply in order to build strong bones and teeth and to avoid the deficiency disease, rickets. Vitamin D is found in oily fish, and to a smaller extent in eggs and full-fat dairy products, but a supplement is the only sure way to ensure an adequate supply for young children. Look for specialised children's supplements or vitamin drops and follow the dosage with care: very young babies are often already prescribed vitamins, so take care not to duplicate. Liquid cod liver oil is an excellent source of vitamin D, but is not normally recommended for very young children because of the

taste and the potential for mistakes in measuring an accurate dosage.

Under fives also have high requirements of iron relative to their body size. Babies are born with a six-month store of iron in their bodies, but breast milk supplies very little, and young children can quickly become deficient. In a Ministry of Agriculture survey, a worrying proportion of the children in the one-and-a-half to four-and-a-half age group were found to have low iron levels – which may lead to lowered IQ and poor concentration.

Deficiency of iron is believed to be on the increase because parents are moving towards 'healthier' diets with less meat. But although it is desirable to reduce the intake of fatty meat sources, some lean red meat or liver in the diet of under fives is very helpful to meet iron needs. For vegetarian children, good iron sources include dried fruit, pulses and broccoli, but these sources should be consumed with some vitamin C (e.g. a glass of orange juice) to improve iron absorption.

TEENAGERS

Emphasis on: calcium, iron, zinc

Teenagers require more calcium than adults to satisfy the demands of their growing bones. The amount consumed during adolescence helps determine bone strength later in life and can lessen the chance of developing osteoporosis. The National Osteoporosis Society recommends that teenagers consume at least 1000 mg calcium a day – an amount that can be obtained through the daily consumption of 600 ml skimmed milk, plus a pot of fruit yoghurt and a small piece of Cheddar cheese. Teenage girls who are pregnant or breastfeeding have even higher requirements, and should ideally consume half as much calcium again, or take a calcium supplement.

adolescent boys and girls need extra iron

Both adolescent boys and girls need extra iron. Good sources include red meat and liver, but the mineral is also found in green leafy vegetables, dried fruit and fortified breakfast cereals. An inadequate intake can lead to poor mental as well as physical performance. High-dose supplements of iron should only be given with a doctor's advice, but a multivitamin with added iron can be given to prevent deficiencies, especially in young girls with heavy periods.

Zinc is important in the development of a healthy reproductive system, and teenagers have increased needs for the mineral. There is some evidence that zinc deficiency is linked with the slimming disease anorexia nervosa, and too little zinc has also been linked with aggressive and delinquent behaviour in teenagers. Additionally, zinc helps maintain a healthy skin, and may even help in cases of acne. Good sources include fish, meat and whole grains. A supplement of up to 15 mg can be taken daily.

WOMEN DURING MENSTRUATION

Emphasis on: iron

Throughout their fertile lives, women need on average almost twice as much of the mineral iron as men. For women with light or moderate periods a healthy diet is normally enough to satisfy these needs, but those with heavy bleeding could benefit from a supplement providing the entire RDA of iron. If you think you might be anaemic (symptoms include pallor, weakness, dizziness, lethargy) don't attempt to self-supplement. See your doctor for a blood test, as higher levels of iron – only available on prescription – may be needed.

MEN AND WOMEN PLANNING A FAMILY

Emphasis on: antioxidants, folic acid

It's hard to believe, but the health of a child can be influenced by the nutritional status of both parents well before birth. If the parents are eating a healthy, balanced diet at the time of conception, their offspring are likely to enjoy better health. By the same token, if both parents are run down or have a poor intake of vitamins and minerals, their children may be more prone to diseases such as heart disease, diabetes and brittle bones later in life.

For men planning to start a family, antioxidants, including vitamin E, vitamin C, zinc and selenium, are essential for fit and healthy sperm. Stepping up the intake of fruits, vegetables and grains will help supply these antioxidants and protect sperm from the type of damage that may increase the risk of a miscarriage or childhood cancers.

Women who are planning babies can also benefit from a healthy diet, but require more folic acid than can be provided through food alone. A 400 μg supplement daily helps reduce the risk of a baby being born with spina bifida and should be taken by any woman who stands a chance of becoming pregnant. It is also important to increase the intake of folic acid from foods such as green leafy vegetables, potatoes and oranges. Look out for the 'F' flash on packaged foods which indicates they have been fortified with the vitamin.

WOMEN DURING PREGNANCY

Emphasis on: B vitamins, vitamin C, vitamin A, iron, calcium, vitamin D, omega-3 fatty acids

Several vitamins and minerals are needed in higher levels during pregnancy. For example more B-complex vitamins are needed to match an increase in energy requirements, and vitamin C is needed in higher amounts for development of the baby's tissues and maintenance of the mother's immune system. In both cases, a healthy diet including whole grains, lean meats, green vegetables and citrus fruits should cover the increased needs.

Vitamin A intake also needs to be stepped up in pregnancy. This can be achieved through eating more red/orange vegetables, dairy products or eggs. Liver is an extremely rich source of vitamin A, but it is not recommended in pregnancy because the high levels of the vitamin may harm the foetus.

Experts are divided about whether needs for iron are increased during pregnancy. The mineral is vital for creating the baby's blood supply and if intakes are insufficient, the mum-to-be can become anaemic. In the USA, it is recommended that all women take an iron supplement during their pregnancy, but in the UK, it is generally felt that increases in the efficiency of iron absorption can cover the extra needs. Whether your doctor advises you to take iron supplements or not, it is important to ensure a good dietary supply of the mineral from sources such as red meat, green vegetables, dried fruit and fortified breakfast cereals.

Pregnant women should also try to increase their intake of bone-building calcium from foods such as cheese, milk and yoghurt. (Unpasteurised dairy products and mould-ripened or blue-vein cheeses shouldn't be eaten during pregnancy because of the risk of listeria infection.) If you dislike or can't tolerate dairy sources of calcium, eat foods such as fortified soya milk, tofu, spinach, canned fish, beans, sesame seeds, dried figs, oranges and white bread. A dietary supply of vitamin D is also essential to aid the absorption of the calcium. Get this from eggs (well-cooked), butter and especially canned fish.

Certain special polyunsaturates, known as omega-3 fatty acids, may be important in ensuring optimal brain development of the unborn child. It is possible to manufacture them from food sources such as green leafy vegetables and linseed, but the crucial needs of pregnancy are best met by eating two to three portions of oily fish a week.

WOMEN WHO ARE BREASTFEEDING

Emphasis on: vitamin A, calcium, B vitamins, zinc
Requirements for vitamin A are increased by over fifty per cent during lactation; the extra can be supplied by a helping of spinach or broccoli, or a portion of mango or cantaloupe melon. The vitamin is also found in full-fat dairy products, and in very large amounts in liver. It is particularly important for infant growth and development.

Calcium requirements are also increased during breastfeeding, as the mineral is diverted into the milk for the baby's developing bones. If dietary intakes are inadequate, calcium will be leached from the mother's own bones to make up the deficit. The additional 550 mg per day required can be supplied by drinking an extra 450 ml of milk.

Extra B vitamins are essential during breastfeeding. If the extra B vitamin requirements are not met, breastfeeding mums may become tired and depressed, and milk production can be affected. The additional B vitamins can be supplied by eating an extra bowl of fortified cereal, such as cornflakes, with skimmed milk. Other good sources of B vitamins include meat, milk, wholemeal bread and potatoes.

Extra B vitamins are essential during breastfeeding

Extra zinc is important for general growth and development and for a healthy immune system in both mother and baby. Low levels in breast milk have been associated with poor infant weight gain. Requirements are virtually doubled in lactation; you can get the extra 6 mg from 100 g lean minced beef or just one oyster!

In theory, simply eating an additional 500 calories or so a day will supply all the extra vitamin and minerals needed by breastfeeding mums. But it's important that these calories are nutritionally dense – i.e. not made entirely of sugary and fatty snack foods which provide largely 'empty' calories. Because many mums are simply too busy to always eat well, a multivitamin and mineral supplement makes a good nutritional safeguard.

WOMEN DURING THE MENOPAUSE

Emphasis on: calcium, magnesium, zinc, manganese, vitamin D
Calcium intakes should be increased at the menopause to compensate for the sudden drop in oestrogen levels. Oestrogen is the main female hormone, and it acts as a bone strengthener during a woman's reproductive years. Hormone replacement therapy (HRT) can help offset the bone loss which may occur after the menopause, but the National Osteoporosis Society recommends that all women also take a 1000 mg calcium supplement to help prevent brittle bones.

There is evidence that other minerals, such as magnesium, zinc and manganese, help reduce losses in bone density when included in a supplement with calcium. Vitamin D is also important, as it helps calcium be better absorbed.

WOMEN AND MEN IN MIDLIFE

Emphasis on: folic acid, vitamin E

Increasing amounts of research are indicating that men in the forty to fifty age group could benefit from extra folic acid, as this vitamin helps lower raised levels of homocysteine – a heart-attack risk factor – in the blood. Many men have a genetic tendency towards high homocysteine levels, so it's well worth them taking a supplement of folic acid just in case.

As heart-attack risk rises in midlife, it is also time that men in particular start thinking about increasing vitamin E intake. A recent study showed that 400–800 IU of the vitamin taken daily (as natural vitamin E capsules)

> *men in the forty to fifty age group could benefit from extra folic acid*

reduced the risk of non-fatal heart attack by seventy-five per cent in middle-aged men with angina.

SENIORS

Emphasis on: vitamin D, B vitamins, antioxidants, potassium

Official figures often suggest that older people actually require less vitamins and minerals due to decreased energy expenditure. But, in practice, requirements may be greater due to less efficient absorption. In particular there is strong evidence that ageing increases the requirements for vitamin D – needed for strong bones and to prevent hip fractures, and certain B vitamins which are particularly important for brain function and energy release. Liver is an excellent food which includes both these nutrients in ample quantities and should ideally be eaten once a week.

Antioxidants (including vitamin C, E, beta carotene and selenium) help protect against abnormal cell changes and other age-related oxidation processes including skin ageing and eye diseases such as macular degeneration and cataracts. Older people should ensure a good intake of antioxidant-rich fruits and vegetables to help combat these diseases. The best choices are deep and brightly coloured fruits and vegetables, which tend to be richest in nutrients. For older people who are unwilling or unable to eat at least five portions of fruits and vegetables a day, a multivitamin or antioxidant supplement can be a good choice.

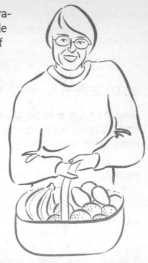

The mineral potassium is vital for everyone's health but it becomes more important in older people because it helps to keep blood pressure normal. Potassium-rich foods are again fruit and vegetables, with particularly good sources being bananas, oranges and avocados.

SMOKERS

Emphasis on: vitamin C, antioxidants

With all the health warnings attached to smoking, no smoker can claim not to know the risk he or she takes. Each puff of smoke contains literally billions of free radicals – unstable molecules that attack and oxidise body cells – and the only way to stop the damage they cause is to quit the evil weed completely.

In the meantime, smokers have increased nutritional needs –

> *smokers have increased nutritional needs*

in particular for vitamin C and other nutritional antioxidants which offset the damaging effects of free radicals. Including a good range of fresh fruit and vegetables in the diet is the best way to meet this increased antioxidant need, but supplements may be a more practical option.

Most authorities recommend that smokers need 80–100 mg extra vitamin C a day just to keep their blood levels the same as non-smokers. That is the amount in one large orange, or about 75 g green pepper.

ATHLETES

Emphasis on: B vitamins, antioxidants, iron

Keen athletes have a greater need for energy and a wide range of nutrients than sedentary individuals. In particular, sportsmen and -women may need more B-complex vitamins to aid energy release in cells, and more antioxidant nutrients (vitamin C, E and beta carotene) to mop up the harmful free radicals produced by large amounts of aerobic exercise.

Foods such as pasta, bread, rice and potatoes are the best ways to supply the extra B-vitamin needs of athletes as they also provide carbohydrates, which are the ideal energy source for working muscles. Most of the extra antioxidants required can be supplied by ensuring an intake of at least five portions of fruits and vegeta-

> *antioxidant nutrients mop up the harmful free radicals produced by large amounts of aerobic exercise*

bles each day, but a daily supplement of vitamin E may also still be desirable, especially for athletes training at a high altitude. (Vitamin E helps the body use the reduced level of oxygen more effectively in this situation.)

Several studies indicate that low levels of ferritin (the main storage form of iron) are common in some groups of athletes. In particular, various stages of iron deficiency have been observed amongst élite athletes. For example in Canada, twenty per cent of the male and eighty-two per cent of the female élite long-distance runners were iron deficient, and thirty-five per cent of a corresponding group in Finland also had low iron levels.

Women athletes are especially at risk because of the increased metabolic demands of heavy exercise coupled with monthly blood loss through menstruation. And both women and men involved in high impact, endurance sports (such as marathon running) are also at risk. Sustained movement in such sports can break down red blood cells and cause tiny intestinal ruptures that lead to minor bleeding and iron loss.

Too much as well as too little iron can cause problems, so the best way for athletes to increase their iron intake is through dietary means (e.g more lean red meat, liver) or through a *modest* supplement.

VEGETARIANS AND VEGANS

Emphasis on: vitamin B12, vitamin D, iron, calcium, iodine
Most nutrients can be supplied adequately by a vegetarian diet, but intake of those which only occur naturally in animal food – such as vitamin B12 (for a healthy nervous system) and vitamin D (for strong bones) – may be marginal. Vitamin B12 can normally be obtained in sufficient amounts from dairy products, but vegans (who avoid dairy products and eggs) may need to supplement, or otherwise eat plenty of foods such as yeast extract, fortified breakfast cereals and fortified soya milk. Vitamin D can be found in vegetable margarines and fortified breakfast cereals.

Contrary to popular belief, most vegetarians and vegans actually consume adequate amounts of iron in their diets. However the absorption of the mineral from vegetable sources is very much poorer than from meat. In practice, vegetarians and vegans adapt to their diet by an increased ability to absorb iron, and their normally higher intake of vitamin C is also useful as this vitamin markedly enhances the uptake of iron from non-meat sources. However vegetarians and vegans should avoid drinking tea with meals, as the tannins in the drink can have an adverse effect on iron absorption.

vegetarians and vegans should avoid drinking tea with meals

Dietary intakes of bone-strengthening calcium are generally no lower in vegetarians than in omnivores, as both groups include dairy products in their diet. However vegans need to increase consumption of vegetable foods rich in calcium (e.g. broccoli, calcium-enriched soya milk) to compensate for their lack of dairy sources.

A further mineral of concern for vegans is iodine, which plays an important role in regulating metabolism. Milk-drinkers can obtain enough iodine, but vegans need to include fortified foods or seaweeds in their diet to ensure an adequate supply.

SLIMMERS

Emphasis on: vitamin A, vitamin D, vitamin E, iron, calcium, zinc

Anyone who reduces the amount of calories they consume is also likely to reduce their vitamin and mineral intake. However female slimmers, especially teenagers, are most at risk. Even on a normal diet of around 2000 calories per day it is not always easy for a woman to get her daily recommended intake of all nutrients. On a low-calorie diet it becomes harder still, and without careful planning, the results can be symptoms such as tiredness and poor skin in the short term, and more serious problems such as brittle bones in the future.

Most likely to be missing are the fat-soluble vitamins A, D and E. This is because slimmers tend to cut out full-fat dairy products and other full-fat foods that normally supply these nutrients. It is possible to substitute vitamin A by eating plenty of deep green and orange/yellow fruits and vegetables, and vitamin D can be made in the skin by exposing it to the sun. However vitamin E can be harder to obtain unless nuts and seeds or vegetable oils are included in the diet.

Iron, calcium and zinc can also be lacking in reduced-calorie diets as slimmers reduce their intake of dairy products and meat. The best safeguard for slimmers is to eat as balanced a diet as possible, but also to supplement with a full-spectrum multivitamin and mineral supplement.

PEOPLE SUFFERING STRESS

Emphasis on: vitamin C, B vitamins

Stress is now a feature of many lifestyles, and represents one of the most damaging influences on health. One of the consequences of stress is an increased need for vitamin C, due to the vitamin being rapidly depleted from the adrenal glands during the production of adrenalin and other stress hormones. People who suffer from chronic stress should make sure they increase their intake of vitamin C-rich foods. A good supply of the vitamin will also help reduce susceptibility to infections, which can be more of a problem when the nervous system is under strain.

Requirements for the B-complex vitamins are also elevated when we experience mental stress. Nervous tissue has a very high requirement for energy and uses up the B vitamins at an increasingly higher rate the more active it becomes.

PEOPLE USING ALCOHOL AND STIMULANTS

Emphasis on: B vitamins, iron

A small amount of alcohol – no more than one or two units (e.g. glasses of wine) daily – can actually boost the immune system and lower cholesterol levels. But excess drinking increases the need for vitamins, particularly thiamin and other B vitamins involved in converting alcohol to energy. Some of the typical symptoms of excess alcohol intake are nervous symptoms (thiamin and B6 deficiency), skin and gastric ailments (riboflavin and niacin deficiency) and anaemia (folic-acid deficiency). It is important that alcoholics and heavy drinkers get a good supplement of B vitamins whilst also taking appropriate steps to drink less. Heavy drinkers may also need more vitamin A, vitamin C and zinc.

Coffee and tea may affect nutrient status

Coffee and tea may also affect nutrient status; they contain stimulants which in excess can interfere with metabolism and marginally increase vitamin need. In addition, tea and coffee can reduce the absorption of certain minerals from food – for example when tea is drunk with a bowl of cereal, the tannins it contains reduce iron absorption by as much as sixty per cent.

WOMEN TAKING THE CONTRACEPTIVE PILL

Emphasis on: folic acid, vitamin C, B vitamins

Women who take oral contraceptives have an increased need for various nutrients; in fact one Australian study showed that no vitamin is entirely unaffected by the pill. In particular, folic acid, vitamin C and vitamin B6 requirements are increased; if vitamin B6 levels are inadequate, the body increasingly relies on the amino acid, tryptophan, to produce it, which in turn can deplete levels of the neurotransmitter serotonin and lead to depression.

Women who take the pill must be especially careful to ensure they receive a healthy and nutritious diet, paying particular attention to foods like fish, lean meat, grains and green vegetables which are rich in the B vitamins and vitamin C. Taking a multivitamin may also be a good precaution.

DRUGS THAT CAN AFFECT YOUR VITAMIN BALANCE

	VITAMINS DEPLETED					
	B Complex	C	A	D	E	K
Painkillers, anti-inflammatory drugs	√(B6)	√				√
Antibiotics	√(most Bs)	√	√		√	√
Diuretics, blood pressure drugs	√(B6, B12 folic acid)	√				
Laxatives			√	√	√	√
Cholesterol-lowering drugs	√(B12, folic acid)		√	√	√	√
Sleeping drugs/ anti-psychotics	√(folic acid)	√	√			√
Gout drugs	√(B2, B12)	√				
Anti-convulsants	√(B6, B12 folic acid)	√		√		√
Digitalis						
Steroids	√(B6)	√		√		

Ca=calcium
Fe=iron
F=fluorine
I=iodine
K=potassium

MINERALS DEPLETED

Ca	Fe	F	I	K	Cu	Mg	Na	P	Zn
			√		√				
√	√			√	√		√		√
√				√		√	√	√	√
√				√			√	√	
√						√		√	
			√		√	√			
	√	√			√	√			
	√								
√				√			√		
√	√						√	√	√

Cu=copper
Mg=magnesium
Na=sodium
P=phosphorus
Zn=zinc

CHAPTER 7

An A–Z of ailments

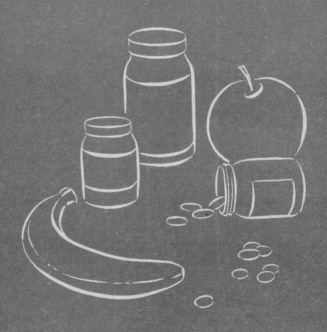

I t is widely accepted that what we eat can have a significant effect on our health and well-being. Vitamins, minerals and other dietary factors all play their roles in preventing or combating illness, and sometimes altering diet and taking appropriate supplements can be a simple way to combat illness. The following few pages give an A–Z guide to those ailments most likely to respond to nutritional help.

ACNE

Acne occurs when sebaceous glands over-secrete oil as a result of hormonal activity. The oil stimulates the growth of infectious bacteria which in turn causes inflammation and proliferation of the cells. The result is blockage of skin pores, blackheads and spots. Contrary to popular opinion too many chocolates or chips do not exacerbate acne, but a deficiency of vitamin A can worsen the condition by encouraging over-proliferation of cells and blockage of the sebaceous glands. Zinc may help in the healing of skin, and there is also some evidence that particular anti-inflammatory fatty acids, of the type found in oily fish, vegetable oils and seeds, may help.

Eat more foods rich in zinc such as lean meat, grains and seafood. Take one or two teaspoons of cod liver oil daily to provide vitamin A and anti-inflammatory fatty acids.

ALLERGIES

Allergies arise when the immune system reacts against a harmless food or substance as if it were a foreign body. For example hay fever is an allergy to pollen, and coeliac disease is an allergy to wheat protein. The only sensible way to deal with the allergic reaction is to avoid the offending food or substance. Increasing the intake of vitamin C can also help, as this vitamin has a mild anti-histamine action. Evening primrose can help some allergic conditions, by damping down an over-active immune system.

Eat more fruit and vegetables for a healthy immune system. Take a 1000 mg vitamin C supplement and 2–3 g evening primrose oil daily.

Avoid trigger foods or environments. Common dietary culprits include milk, wheat, eggs, fish, shellfish, nuts, soya beans and additives.

ARTHRITIS

Arthritis can affect people of all ages. There are two types: rheumatoid arthritis, which involves a fault in the immune system; and osteoarthritis, which is caused by simple wear and tear on the joints. In both cases there is inflammation, and increasing the intake of antioxidant-rich foods and oily fish rich in anti-inflammatory fatty acids can help. Research also indicates that vitamin D may ease some of the symptoms of osteoarthritis.

Eat more fruits and vegetables rich in antioxidants and take one to two teaspoons of cod liver oil daily. Rheumatoid arthritis sufferers could also try taking 100–200 μg selenium daily.

Avoid fatty red meats, full-fat dairy products and other sources of saturated fats that may encourage inflammation in the body.

ASTHMA

Asthma is an allergic condition which causes constriction of the airways and (sometimes severe) difficulty in breathing. Dietary measures that may help include regular consumption of oily fish which encourages the production of anti-inflamma-

> *Eating more magnesium found in leafy green vegetables, grains and nuts can relax the airways*

tory chemicals in the body and a diet rich in antioxidants which help mop up the harmful free radicals produced as a part of the inflammatory process. Eating more magnesium found in leafy green vegetables, grains and nuts can also relax the airways. If your attacks are stress related, step up your intake of pulses, grains and lean meat as they supply B vitamins vital for the nervous system.

Eat more fruits and vegetables, oily fish, green vegetables, nuts and grains. Try taking a supplement of fish oils and/or evening primrose oil.

Avoid foods that might provoke an attack. These vary from person to person, but can include cow's milk, sulphite additives and wine.

BRUISES, BURNS AND CUTS

Nobody escapes the occasional minor injury, but with a healthy diet and the right vitamins and minerals it is possible to heal more quickly. In particular, stepping up the intake of vitamin C, zinc and vitamin E will help. Bioflavonoids, found in fruits such as oranges, cherries and grapes, can help strengthen capillaries and reduce the risk of bruising.

Eat more fruits and vegetables and foods rich in zinc such as lean meat, grains and seafood. Take 500 mg vitamin C with added bioflavonoids twice a day; also an antioxidant or multivitamin supplement providing vitamin E and zinc.

CARPAL TUNNEL SYNDROME

This is a painful condition involving inflammation of the nerves as they pass through the wrist. In severe cases an operation is needed to relieve pressure on the nerves, but some studies have shown that high doses of vitamin B6 can resolve the problem before it gets this severe.

Take 50–200 mg vitamin B6 daily. Many nutritional practitioners recommend that this dosage of vitamin B6 should also be accompanied by a B complex.

CRAMP

Cramp is a condition in which muscles go into spasm and contract painfully. It can often wake sufferers at night. Calcium- and magnesium-rich foods help muscles to function normally and may reduce the incidence of cramp.

Eat more low-fat dairy products, grains, green vegetables and nuts. Try drinking a milky drink before bed, and taking a calcium and magnesium supplement.

CIRCULATION PROBLEMS

Poor circulation can manifest itself in cold hands and feet and may exacerbate symptoms of nerve damage in diabetics. Allium (onion family) vegetables contain sulphur compounds that can help reduce the stickiness of the blood, and particular long-chain fatty acids found in marine foods also help thin the blood and improve circulation. A number of 'warming' herbs also help stimulate blood flow.

Eat more garlic, ginger and oily fish. Taking a supplement of the herb ginkgo biloba can also help.

    Avoid too many saturated fats (in foods such as fatty meats) that can lead to more 'sticky' blood.

COLDS AND FLU

Everyone gets colds and flu from time to time, but frequent suffering may indicate the immune stem is over-stressed. Step up your intake of vitamin A-rich foods which maintain healthy mucous passages, and eat more zinc to help boost the immune system and reduce the risk of succumbing to infection. Vitamin C (citrus fruits and juices), garlic and beta carotene-rich foods can all also help.

> *Suck zinc lozenges and take 1000–2000mg vitamin C per day when you feel a cold coming on*

Eat more fruits and vegetables (especially brightly coloured varieties, onions and garlic), citrus fruits, grains, lean meat and oily fish. Suck zinc lozenges and take 1000–2000 mg vitamin C per day when you feel a cold coming on.

DEPRESSION

Mild depression can result from many factors, and poor diet may be one of them. Carbohydrate-rich and vitamin B6-rich foods can raise the levels of the anti-depressive chemical serotonin in the brain.

Eat more dried fruit, pasta, rice and bread. Bananas and nuts also include vitamin B6 which can help depression associated with use of the contraceptive pill or premenstruation. For mild to moderate depression, a supplement of St John's wort may also help.

ECZEMA

Eczema is a skin condition thought often to result from an abnormal immune response. Diets rich in oily fish may help to combat some of the inflammation, and evening primrose oil can also improve the condition in some people. Zinc supplements aid healing.

Eat more oily fish, fresh foods and vegetables. Take at least 2–3 g evening primrose oil daily and 15 mg zinc.

FATIGUE

Fatigue may be caused by several factors – ranging from too many late nights to hormonal changes or anaemia. One of the most common nutritional causes is iron deficiency, although a deficiency of the B vitamins can play a role as well.

Eat more sources of iron and B vitamins such as lean red meat and liver to provide anaemia-preventive iron and B vitamins. Vegetarians should increase their intake of green leafy vegetables and whole grains.

Avoid drinking lots of coffee in an attempt to feel less tired. Excess caffeine stimulates the adrenal glands, and in the long term depletes energy levels by causing fluctuating blood sugar levels.

HEART DISEASE

Heart disease is one of the biggest killers in the UK and poor diet is mainly to blame. High levels of saturated fats raise cholesterol levels, whilst too much salt causes high blood pressure in susceptible individuals. On the plus side, a diet rich in antioxidants, especially vitamin E, can prevent cholesterol becoming oxidised (the precursor to it clogging the arteries), and oily fish provides fatty acids which thin the blood and reduce the risk of thrombosis. Garlic is beneficial for heart health and selenium may also reduce the incidence of cardiovascular disease. New research indicates that taking a folic acid supplement can be useful because it lowers the levels of homocysteine – a heart-disease risk factor – in the blood.

Eat more fruits and vegetables, oily fish, unsalted nuts and seeds, olive oil and garlic. Take a 200–400 mg vitamin E supplement, and a 400 μg folic acid supplement.

Avoid saturated fats (found mainly in animal products) and salty foods which can raise blood cholesterol and blood pressure.

HIGH BLOOD PRESSURE

High blood pressure leads to many heart attacks and strokes that could otherwise have been prevented. The main dietary measures needed to tackle high blood pressure involve reducing salt (sodium) intake and losing any excess weight. However there is evidence that a diet rich in potassium and magnesium can also help.

Eat more potassium-rich foods. These include all fruits and vegetables, but particularly dried fruit, bananas, avocados, potatoes and oranges. Increase the intake of magnesium from green leafy vegetables, pulses and whole grains.

Avoid excess sodium (salt) added to many processed products. Don't add salt at the table.

INFERTILITY

Infertility affects as many as one in six couples. If there is not a physical cause, improving diet may help. For example zinc – found in foods such as seafood, lean meat and grains – is required for the health of both male and female reproductive organs and a deficiency may result in low sperm levels or a low birth-weight baby. Vitamin E-rich foods such as avocados, vegetable oils and nuts can also protect sperm function, as can selenium.

> *Vitamin E-rich foods such as avocados, vegetable oils and nuts can protect sperm function*

Eat more fruits and vegetables, nuts and seeds, and take a good antioxidant formulation providing zinc, selenium and vitamin E (males and females).

KIDNEY STONES

Kidney stones are caused by the painful crystallisation of calcium oxalate in the kidney. Contrary to popular opinion, calcium-rich foods actually reduce the risk of suffering a kidney stone. Vitamin B6 and magnesium can also reduce the risk of a stone forming.

Eat more, not less, foods rich in calcium (dairy products, pulses, green vegetables). Eat foods rich in vitamin B6 such as fish, bananas, nuts and liver. Take a supplement providing magnesium. Drink plenty of water.

Avoid foods rich in oxalic acid, e.g. rhubarb, chocolate, spinach, beetroot. Don't take calcium in supplement form.

MIGRAINES

Migraines can have many causes, but food can have a bearing on how many of these painful headaches you suffer.

Eat more magnesium-rich foods such as green vegetables, dried fruit, grains, etc. which help relax the muscles in the head.

Avoid trigger foods such as cheese, coffee and red wine (they vary from person to person).

MOUTH ULCERS

Mouth ulcers can occur as a result of cuts, bites or chafing in the mouth, but are also often stress related. A deficiency of B vitamins can sometimes trigger the condition.

Eat more B complex-rich foods such as grains, milk, meat, pulses. Also take a multivitamin supplement providing B vitamins and zinc for healing.

Avoid too many acid or citrus foods which may make ulcers more painful.

OSTEOPOROSIS

Osteoporosis is a bone-thinning disease which affects one in three women after the menopause and an increasing number of men. The disease is better prevented than treated, because once the symptoms appear, a lot of the bone mass has already been lost. Weight-bearing exercise, e.g. walking and jogging, can build bone mass early in life, and prevent loss later on; hormone replacement therapy after the menopause is another option. The main dietary measures that help are a high intake of calcium and vitamin D. There is also evidence that minerals such as zinc, magnesium, manganese, boron and copper also enhance the strength of bones.

Eat more calcium-rich foods including dairy products, watercress, spring greens, broccoli and nuts. Take 1000 mg calcium with vitamin D, plus a multi-mineral supplement.

Avoid too much salt, alcohol and phosphoric acid (found in cola and some other fizzy drinks), as these can leach calcium from the bones.

PREMENSTRUAL SYNDROME

Premenstrual syndrome (PMS) is a collection of physical and emotional symptoms suffered by women in the days approaching a period. Consuming regular amounts of carbohydrate foods helps keep blood-sugar levels constant and eases symptoms. Evening primrose oil can also help some women because it provides fatty acids that influence hormone balance in a positive way. Vitamin B6 and magnesium also help by nourishing the nervous system.

Eat more regular snacks rich in carbohydrates, vitamin B6 and magnesium (good choices include bananas, dried fruit and nuts). Take 2–3 g evening primrose oil in the two weeks leading up to a period.

PROSTATE TROUBLES

Lots of men get prostate troubles as they get older. All men who experience difficulty with urination should see a doctor, but consuming more of certain nutrients may also be useful. For example the prostate gland is very rich in zinc, and increasing the intake of the mineral seems to help slow down the development of benign prostate disease. Certain essential fatty acids can also help, as does a herb called saw palmetto.

Eat more whole grains, fish, lean meat, nuts and seeds. Take 15 mg zinc, 2–3 g evening primrose oil and a supplement of saw palmetto daily.

PSORIASIS

Psoriasis is a debilitating skin condition in which the skin is reddened and forms scales. Exposure to sunlight can help, as can reducing stress levels. Vitamin D supplements have been reported to help some patients, but most helpful are fish oils which sooth the skin because they contain anti-inflammatory fatty acids.

Eat more oily fish and take one or two teaspoons of cod liver oil daily (provides vitamin D as well as anti-inflammatory fatty acids).

CHAPTER 8

Quiz: Are you getting enough?

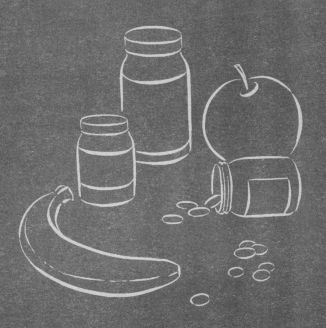

The more balanced and varied your diet, the less your chance of suffering vitamin and mineral deficiencies. The following quiz is designed to give you a rough idea of how vitamin- and mineral-rich your diet is, and which micronutrients, if any, you may be lacking.

If guidance on portion sizes is required, see 'The balance of good health' in chapter one.

Question one

a Do you eat less than one portion per day of liver / oily fish / red, yellow or leafy green vegetables?

b Do you have less than one portion a day of full-fat dairy products?

Question two

a Do you eat less than one portion of bread / pasta / rice / cereals / pulses per day?

b Do you have less than two portions of meat / liver / eggs per day?

c Are your main meals often eaten in canteens or restaurants?

Question three

a Do you have less than two or three portions of fruit a day?

b Do you eat at least two or three portions of lightly cooked or raw vegetables a day?

c Are your main meals often eaten in canteens or restaurants?

d Do you smoke?

Question four

a Do you avoid using butter and butter substitutes?

b Do you have less than one portion of fortified breakfast cereal / oily fish / eggs per day?

c Do you spend only a little time outside in sunlight?

Question five

a Do you have less than two slices of bread per day?

b Do you have less than one portion of red meat / fortified breakfast cereal / liver / dried fruit / pulses / deep green vegetables per day?

c Do you have three or less portions of fresh fruit and vegetables / fruit juice a day?

Question six

a Do you have less than two portions of dairy produce / canned fish with bones (e.g. sardines) a day?

b Do you eat white bread or green leafy vegetables only occasionally?

c Have you answered yes to more than one question in five?

Question seven

a Do you eat meat / liver / cereals and grains / seafood / pulses very infrequently?

b Do you try to eat a lot of fibre, e.g. always choose wholemeal varieties of bread, pasta and rice, and have whole-wheat breakfast cereals?

Now see how you match up:

Question one

If you answered yes to either a or b, you may be short of vitamin A. This risk is increased if you answered yes to both.

What you can do: Increase your intake of dairy products (look for low-fat milk fortified with vitamins A and D), liver, or sources rich in beta carotene such as carrots, dark green leafy vegetables or tomatoes. Vitamin A is needed to maintain healthy skin and it helps vision in dim light.

Question two

If you answered yes to a, b or c, you may be short of some of the group of twelve B vitamins. The risk is increased if you answered yes to two or more of these.

What you can do: Increase your intake of fortified breakfast cereals, offal, wholemeal products, yeast extract, pulses and dairy products. The B-complex vitamins are easily destroyed by cooking, so food in canteens and restaurants may be low in these vitamins. B vitamins are important for the release of energy from food, overall well-being and healthy hair and skin.

Question three

If you answered yes to a, b, c or d, you may be short of vitamin C. The risk is increased if you answered yes to two or more of these.

What you can do: Increase your intake of fresh fruit (particularly citrus fruit), juices, tomatoes and fresh and frozen vegetables. Try to eat as much freshly prepared food as possible; prolonged cooking and standing can destroy the vitamins. Vitamin C is required for healthy skin and gums, and for building up resistance to infection. It also aids the absorption of iron.

Question four

If you answered yes to a, b or c, you may be short in vitamin D. This risk is increased if you answered yes to more than one of these.

What you can do: The action of sunlight on the skin is the easiest way to boost your vitamin-D intake. But if you don't manage to get out in the sun much, you should eat oily fish, eggs and a little butter. Vitamin D works with calcium and phosphorus to build and maintain strong bones.

Question five

If you answered yes to a, b or c, you may be short of iron. This risk is increased if you answered yes to more than one of these. *What you can do*: Increase your levels of iron by boosting your intake of dried fruit, nuts or pulses and small portions of red meat, especially liver. Iron is a mineral, and absorption is increased by vitamin-C intake, so ensure you are eating plenty of the foods mentioned in the answers to question three.

Question six

If you answered yes to a, b or c, you may be short of calcium. This risk is increased if you answered yes to more than one of these.
What you can do: Increase your intake of reduced-fat milk and cheese, eggs, leafy vegetables, canned pilchards and sardines. Vegans and non-dairy eaters should eat plenty of pulses, nuts, dried fruit and cereals. Calcium, in conjunction with phosphorus and vitamin D, is needed to build strong bones and teeth. A good intake in early life is important as this is when calcium is laid down in the bones.

Question seven

If you answered yes to either a or b, you could be short of zinc. *What you can do*: Increase your levels of zinc by boosting your intake of pulses, grains, small portions of meat and liver, seafood (particularly crab meat and oysters). Zinc is important in maintaining healthy skin and is essential for normal growth and reproduction.

(Quiz questions courtesy of Boots)

APPENDIX – CONVERSION TABLE

1 litre (l) = 1.76 pints

28 grams (g) = 1 ounce (oz)

1 kilogram (kg) = 2.2 pounds (lb)

approx 5 millilitres (ml)
  = $\frac{1}{8}$ fluid ounce (fl oz) = 1 teaspoon

approx 10 millilitres (ml)
  = $\frac{1}{4}$ fluid ounce (fl oz) = 1 dessertspoon

approx 15 millilitres (ml)
  = $\frac{1}{2}$ fluid ounce (fl oz) = 1 tablespoon

1 g = 1/1000 kg

1 mg = 1/1000 g

1 microgram (mcg or μg) = 1/1000 mg

- ☐ **Apples & Pears** £3.99
  GLORIA THOMAS
  0 75281 604 7

- ☐ **Arousing Aromas** £3.99
  KAY COOPER
  0 75281 546 6

- ☐ **Body Foods For Women**
  £6.99
  JANE CLARKE
  0 75280 922 9

- ☐ **Coping With Your Premature Baby** £4.99
  PENNY STANWAY
  0 75281 596 2

- ☐ **Cranks Recipe Book** £6.99
  CRANKS RESTAURANTS
  1 85797 140 X

- ☐ **Eat Safely** £3.99
  JANET WRIGHT
  0 75281 544 X

- ☐ **Entertaining with Cranks** £6.99
  CRANKS RESTAURANTS
  0 75282 579 8

- ☐ **Food** £6.99
  SUSAN POWTER
  0 75280 315 8

- ☐ **The Good Mood Guide** £4.99
  ROS & JEREMY HOLMES
  0 75282 584 4

- ☐ **Harmonise Your Home** £4.99
  GRAHAM GUNN
  0 75281 665 9

- ☐ **Health Spa at Home** £3.99
  JOSEPHINE FAIRLEY
  0 75281 545 8

- ☐ **Juice Up Your Energy Levels** £3.99
  LESLEY WATERS
  0 75281 602 0

- ☐ **Kitchen Pharmacy** £7.99
  ROSE ELLIOT & CARLO DE PAOLI
  0 75281 725 6

- ☐ **A Natural History of the Senses** £7.99
  DIANE ACKERMAN
  1 85799 403 5

- ☐ **The Natural Way To Stop Snoring** £4.99
  DR ELIZABETH SCOTT
  0 75280 067 1

- ☐ **The New Cranks Recipe Book** £6.99
  NADINE ABENSUR
  0 75281 677 2

- ☐ **Sensitive Skin** £4.99
  JOSEPHINE FAIRLEY
  0 75281 547 4

- ☐ **Spring Clean Your System**
  JANE GARTON £3.99
  0 75281 601 2

- ☐ **Stop the Insanity!** £6.99
  SUSAN POWTER
  1 85797 323 2

- ☐ **Vegetarian Slimming** £6.99
  ROSE ELLIOT
  0 75280 173 2

All Orion/Phoenix titles are available at your local bookshop or from the following address:

> Littlehampton Book Services
> Cash Sales Department L
> 14 Eldon Way, Lineside Industrial Estate
> Littlehampton
> West Sussex BN17 7HE
> *telephone* 01903 721596, *facsimile* 01903 730914

Payment can either be made by credit card (Visa and Mastercard accepted) or by sending a cheque or postal order made payable to *Littlehampton Book Services*.
DO NOT SEND CASH OR CURRENCY.

Please add the following to cover postage and packing

UK and BFPO:
£1.50 for the first book, and 50p for each additional book to a maximum of £3.50

Overseas and Eire:
£2.50 for the first book plus £1.00 for the second book and 50p for each additional book ordered

- -

BLOCK CAPITALS PLEASE

name of cardholder	*delivery address*
....	*(if different from cardholder)*
address of cardholder	....
....	....
....	....
....	....
postcode	*postcode* ....

☐ I enclose my remittance for £..............................

☐ please debit my Mastercard/Visa (delete as appropriate)

card number ☐☐☐☐☐☐☐☐☐☐☐☐☐☐☐☐☐

expiry date ☐☐☐☐

signature ....

prices and availability are subject to change without notice